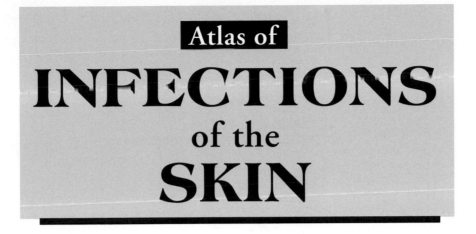

Atlas of
INFECTIONS
of the
SKIN

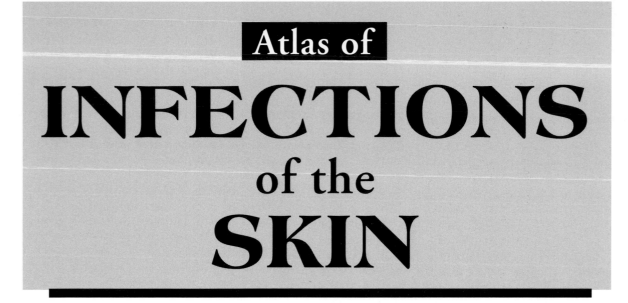

Atlas of
INFECTIONS
of the
SKIN

RAZA ALY, MPH, PhD
Professor of Dermatology, Microbiology-Immunology
University of California San Francisco
San Francisco, California

HOWARD I. MAIBACH, MD
Professor of Dermatology
University of California San Francisco
San Francisco, California

CHURCHILL LIVINGSTONE

A Division of Harcourt Brace & Company

New York, Edinburgh, London, Madrid, Melbourne, San Francisco, Tokyo

CHURCHILL LIVINGSTONE
A Division of Harcourt Brace & Company

The Curtis Center
Independence Square West
Philadelphia, Pennsylvania 19106

Library of Congress Catalogue Card Number—98–074079

ATLAS OF INFECTIONS OF THE SKIN

Copyright © 1999 by Churchill Livingstone   ISBN 0-443-05587-4

Churchill Livingstone® is a registered trademark of Harcourt Brace & Company

™ ⩔ is a trademark of Harcourt Brace & Company.

Printed in the United States of America.

Last digit is the print number: 9 8 7 6 5 4 3 2 1

Contributors

Raza Aly, MPH, PhD

Professor of Dermatology, Microbiology-Immunology, University of California, San Francisco, San Francisco, California

Laboratory Mycology; Superficial Mycoses and Dermatophytoses; Staphylococcal Infections; Streptococcal Infections

Bernard W. Berger, MD

Clinical Assistant Professor of Dermatology, State University of New York at Stony Brook, Stony Brook, New York

Lyme Disease

Timothy G. Berger, MD

Associate Clinical Professor, University of California San Francisco, San Francisco, California

Skin Infections in the Immunocompromised Patient

Karl R. Beutner, MD, PhD

Associate Clinical Professor, Department of Dermatology, University of California San Francisco, San Francisco, California

Antiviral Therapy for Cutaneous Viral Infections

Mary M. Christian, MD

Resident in Dermatology, University of Texas Medical Branch, Galveston, Texas

Human Papillomavirus Infection

John Thorne Crissey, MD

Clinical Professor of Medicine (Dermatology), University of Southern California School of Medicine; Attending Dermatologist, LAC-USC Medical Center, Los Angeles County, Los Angeles, California

Cutaneous Manifestations of Deep Mycoses: Thermally Dimorphic Fungi

Piet De Doncker, MSc, PhD

Associate Director, Clinical Research, Department of Dermatology, Infectious Disease and Allergy, Janssen Research Foundation, Beerse, Belgium

Management and Therapy for Cutaneous Fungal Infection

Mervyn L. Elgart, MD
Clinical Professor of Dermatology, Medicine and Pediatrics, The George Washington University School of Medicine; Attending Physician, George Washington University Hospital; Children's Hospital National Medical Center; Washington Hospital Center, Washington, DC

Subcutaneous Mycoses: Mycetoma, Chromoblastomycoses, Sporotrichosis

Tanya Y. Evans, MD
Clinical Research Fellow in Dermatology, University of Texas Medical Branch, Galveston, Texas

Human Papillomavirus Infection

Jan Faergemann, MD, PhD
Associate Professor, University of Gothenburg; Associate Professor, Sahlgrenska University Hospital, Gothenburg, Sweden

Other Cutaneous Yeast Infections

Ilona J. Frieden, MD
Clinical Professor of Dermatology and Pediatrics, University of California San Francisco, San Francisco, California

Viral Exanthems

Donald L. Greer, PhD
Professor of Clinical Mycology, Departments of Dermatology, Pathology, Microbiology, Louisiana State University Medical Center; Director, Mycology and TB Diagnostic Laboratories, Medical Center of Louisiana at New Orleans, New Orleans, Louisiana

Mycobacterial Infections

Aditya K. Gupta, MD, FRCP
Associate Professor, Department of Dermatology, Division of Medicine, University of Toronto, Toronto, Ontario, Canada

Superficial Mycoses and Dermatophytoses

Joy D. Jester, MD
Clinical Associate Professor, Department of Dermatology, Louisiana State University Medical Center, New Orleans, Louisiana

Varicella-Zoster Virus Infections

Howard I. Maibach, MD
Professor of Dermatology, University of California San Francisco, San Francisco, California

Ectoparasitic Infestations

Michael R. McGinnis, PhD
Department of Pathology, University of Texas Medical Branch, Associate Director, Center for Tropical Diseases; Director, Medical Mycology Research Center, University of Texas Medical Branch, Galveston, Texas

Laboratory Mycology

Lee T. Nesbitt, Jr, MD

Henry Jolly Professor and Chairman of Dermatology, Department of Dermatology, Louisiana State University Medical Center, New Orleans, Louisiana

Mycobacterial Infections; Varicella-Zoster Virus Infections

William C. Noble, PhD, DSc, FRCPath

Professor of Microbiology, University of London; St John's Institute of Dermatology, St Thomas' Hospital, London, United Kingdom

Corynebacterial Infections

Milton Orkin, MD

Clinical Professor, University of Minnesota Medical School, Minneapolis, Minnesota

Ectoparasitic Infestations

Gerald E. Piérard, MD, PhD

Professor, University of Liege; Chairman, University Medical Hospital Sart Tilman, Liege, Belgium

Management and Therapy for Cutaneous Fungal Infection

Charles G. Prober, MD

Professor of Pediatrics, Medicine, Microbiology, and Immunology; Associate Chair, Department of Pediatrics, Stanford University School of Medicine, Stanford, California

Herpesvirus Infections

David T. Roberts, MB, ChB, FRCP (Glasg)

Honorary Clinical Senior Lecturer, University of Glasgow; Consultant Dermatologist, Southern General Hospital, Gaslgow, Scotland

Candidiasis: Cutaneous and Systemic Infections

Stephen K. Tyring, MD, PhD

Professor of Dermatology, Microbiology, Immunology and Internal Medicine, University of Texas Medical Branch, Galveston, Texas

Human Papillomavirus Infection

Guy F. Webster, MD, PhD

Associate Professor of Dermatology, Associate Professor of Internal Medicine, Thomas Jefferson Medical College, Philadelphia, Pennsylvania

Gram-Negative Infections: Folliculitis, Toe Web, Others

Preface

This atlas of skin infection provides guidelines to clinicians and health workers for the early recognition of skin diseases. The cutaneous manifestation of infectious diseases are grouped into bacterial, fungal, viral and parasitic infections. Each disease is discussed using photographs, specific descriptions of skin morphology, a brief mention of the pathology, and an outline of the features of the disease that might prove to be helpful in establishing a diagnosis and appropriate therapy. The differential diagnosis stresses look-alike cutaneous manifestations. Fungal, bacterial, and viral skin infections are among the most common cutaneous afflictions in AIDS patients. Recognition of these patterns of infection should lead rapidly to the correct diagnosis and improved management. The treatments and dosages of all drugs in this atlas have been recommended in medical literature and are in accordance with the practices of the general medical community. Some of the treatments described may not necessarily have specific approval by the Food and Drug Administration for a particular disease. The package insert for each drug should be consulted for use and dosage as approved.

The authors who have contributed to this book are major authorities in their respective fields. We are grateful for their efforts.

RAZA ALY
HOWARD I. MAIBACH

Contents

CHAPTER 1

Laboratory Mycology

Michael R. McGinnis

Raza Aly

SUMMARY

Laboratory Evaluation   Vital for the accurate diagnosis and management of dermatophytosis, dermatomycosis, and yeast infections

Specimen Collections   Skin, scalp, nail

Specimen Evaluation   Direct microscopy

Isolation of Etiologic Agents   Culture of sample

Identification   Yeasts and molds

Information gained from laboratory studies contributes critical information for the diagnosis and management of dermatophytosis, dermatomycosis, and yeast infections. Dermatophytosis is an infection involving hair, nail, or skin on the living host that is caused by fungi classified in the genera *Trichophyton, Microsporum,* or *Epidermophyton.* Infection is characterized by the invasion and multiplication of one of these fungi in tissues. When there is functional or structural damage present with associated signs and symptoms, the condition is a disease. This is in contrast to colonization and contamination, when a fungus innocuously grows on the surface or rests on the surface of hair, nail, or skin. Dermatomycosis in contrast to dermatophytosis is colonization or infection of hair, nail, or skin on the living host that is caused by a fungus other than a dermatophyte. All dermatophytes are classified in the genera *Trichophyton, Microsporum,* and *Epidermophyton,* but all fungi that are classified in these genera are not dermatophytes.

In tissue, nondermatophytes may form hyphae similar to those formed by dermatophytes. They tend, however, to be larger in diameter, less delicate in appearance, more irregular in shape and size, and in some instances dematiaceous. Many filamentous fungi have been described as etiologic agents of dermatomycosis. Cultivation in the laboratory is required for identification.

Yeast infections have been classified under the umbrella term of dermatomycosis by some clinicians. Most people consider yeast infections as a separate entity. The two most common yeast pathogens associated with the cutaneous barriers of the body are *Candida albicans* and *Malassezia furfur;* infections caused by these fungi are referred to as candidiasis and pityriasis versicolor, respectively. Terms like *tinea versicolor* should not be used because the term *tinea* is reserved exclusively for infections caused by dermatophytes.

The principal laboratory contributions to the differential diagnosis and subsequent management of the dermatophytosis consist of the direct microscopic examination of hair, nail, and skin and the isolation and identification of the etiologic agent causing the infection. Laboratory information allows the physician to select the optimal therapeutic drug, its dosage, and the duration of therapy.

SPECIMEN COLLECTION

The quality and quantity of the clinical specimen being used for laboratory examination have direct bearing on the differential diagnosis and subsequent management of the infection. Direct microscopic examination of hair, nail, skin, and their culture helps to determine if a fungal infection is present. Collect as much clinical material as possible so that it may be properly examined. To avoid confusion, cotton balls and swabs should not be used to clean the sites to be sampled or to collect the material for direct microscopic examination and culture. If cotton balls are used to clean the collection site, cotton fibers are typically left behind and can be confused with fungal hyphae during direct microscopic examination. Cotton swabs are also unacceptable for collecting clinical specimens, as specimens may become entangled in the cotton fibers and lost for examination. An exception is the collection of material from moist exudate associated with yeast infections. The large numbers of yeast cells typically present in exudates, such as *C. albicans,* can be readily recovered on the isolation medium.

Collection sites and methods are included in Table 1.1. The collection site must be cleaned prior to sampling to remove grease, oil, topical materials, and microorganisms that are potential contaminants. Seventy percent ethanol in a gauze pad is an excellent cleaning agent. Sterile saline or sterile distilled water can also be used, especially if yeast infections are present in which the application of 70% ethanol may cause discomfort.

Skin

Specimens of fungi located within hair, nail, and skin are collected with a blunt tool such as the edge of a microscope slide or a #15 scalpel blade. The blunt tool dislodges the clinical material containing the fungus. The edge of skin lesions is sampled rather than the central area. The actively growing hyphae are at the

Table 1.1 Specimen Collection

SPECIMEN TYPE	SPECIMEN COLLECTION	
	ACCEPTABLE	UNACCEPTABLE
Hair	Clean[a] area of alopecia	Long hairs or hair clippings
	Scrape scales and black dots; epilate broken hairs and fluorescent hair stubs	<10–12 hairs
	Undersurface of adherent scutula	
Skin		
Scaling lesions	Clean area; scrape scales from advancing edge	Scrapings from central clearing area of lesion, macerated interdigital tissue
Vesicular lesions	Clean lesions; remove portion of vesicle roof	Vesicle fluid or scrapings from the vesicle base
Pityriasis versicolor lesions	Clean lesion; press cellophane tape to lesions	
	Clean lesions; scrape scales from advancing edge	
Interdigital spaces	Clean and remove dried exudate; scrape both sides and base; if fissuring present, scalpel only	Macerated interdigital tissue
	Sample 4th interspace of both feet	
Biopsy	Place between two moistened gauze squares in Petri dish	
	Punch biopsy placed in small tube of sterile saline or water	
Nail		
Superficial	Clean nail surface; remove white, chalky material from nail surface with scalpel	Nail clippings
Deep	Scrape nail bed and underside of nail plate with a curet	Outermost layers of distal subungual debris are undesirable because of heavy saprophyte contamination and greatly diminished viability of fungal pathogens that might be present
	Scrape through surface of nail plate; discard superficial material	
	Collect specimen from deep nail plate	
Paronychial exudate	Scrape and examine for yeasts	

[a] Clean with 70% ethanol in gauze pad; do not use cotton balls or swabs. Collect specimens with a moist gauze pad rubbed on scalp, glass microscope slide, hairbrush, or disposable toothbrush; touch medium in Petri plate to the scalp lesion may be used.

border of the lesions. In the central area, where healing has occurred, the fungus has typically been destroyed (Fig. 1.1).

Portions of the specimen may be collected directly onto the isolation medium, the remaining part being used for preparing the clinical material for direct microscopic examination. Specimens may be collected and placed between two clean glass microscope slides, which are then wrapped in paper or placed in a small clean envelope, such as those used for pills, or onto a piece of clean paper. If the clean paper is composed of both black and white portions, the clinical specimen can be seen more easily, especially against the black background. Even though empty plastic Petri dishes can be used, they are not recommended because there is typically a static electrical charge that makes handling of the clinical material difficult.

The principal infections involving skin are caused by dermatophytes, *M. furfur, C. albicans,* and to a lesser extent other fungi. *M. furfur* is a lipophilic yeast that can be cultured when it is provided with a medium containing an olive oil supplement. The clinical presentation of pityriasis versicolor and the morphology of the pathogen in the stratum corneum are usually diagnostic, and so the culture of the etiologic agent is not generally performed. Cellophane tape can be pressed onto the lesion to collect skin material for direct microscopic examination. Skin scrapings collected in the same manner as for dermatophyte-infected material works well for pityriasis versicolor (Fig. 1.2).

Scalp

Lesions involving the scalp provide two types of clinical material, hair and skin. Material from infections involving the skin are collected in the same manner as from other body sites. In addition to a blunt collecting tool, hairbrushes, toothbrushes, and moistened gauze pads have also been successfully used, especially in children. These types of collection tools can provide material for both direct microscopy and culture. For culture, the brushes and gauze are simply touched on the surface of the isolation medium (Fig. 1.3). Some physicians prefer to press the isolation medium in a Petri dish directly to the scalp lesions.

If hairs fluoresce when exposed to the ultraviolet light from Wood's lamp, they can be selectively plucked for examination. Forceps can be used to collect the fluorescent hairs. Hair clippings are undesirable. If *Trichophyton tonsurans* is the suspected etiologic agent, infected hairs have usually broken off at the skin surface. A scalpel may be required to dig out and collect the hair stubs.

Nail

Of the specimens for dermatologic evaluation, nail material provides the most unique challenges. The differentiation between etiologic agent and saprophytic fungi known to be recoverable from healthy nails without disease can be difficult. The direct microscopic examination and its correlation to what is recovered in culture, or what is not recovered, are important for reaching a diagnosis.

Large portions of nail must be pulverized to increase the surface area of the specimen, which greatly augments the probability of recovering clinically important fungi. The larger the amount of surface area contacting the isolation medium, the greater the opportunity for fungal elements to grow on the medium. In addition, the microscopic examination of the material is enhanced because the specimen can be more effectively cleared with potassium hydroxide, making visualization of the fungal elements easier. Small fragments of the specimens lay flatter in the preparation, contributing to the easier recognition of fungal elements.

Large pieces of nail can be broken down into manageable fragments by using either a nail micronizer or hammer. If a hammer is used, the large nail pieces are placed in a strong bag and struck. A micronizer is a useful tool to pulverize nail samples (Fig. 1.4). For distal subungual onychomycosis, clip the abnormal nail as proximally as possible. The nail bed and underside of the nail plate are scraped with a curette (1 mm). The outermost layers should be discarded because of contamination.

SPECIMEN EXAMINATION

Clinical specimens are examined microscopically for several reasons (Fig. 1.5). First, the presence or absence of fungal elements provides important immediate information useful in the differential diagnosis. Second, the type or types of fungal elements such as hyphae, pseudohyphae, and yeast cells and the presence or absence of melanin provide important information about the identity of the etiologic agent. This information can be used to determine if more than one fungus is contributing to the infection. Third, based on the clinical presentation and probable etiologic agent, an appropriate antifungal agent can be selected and used for therapy. Fourth, information from the direct microscopic examination may suggest modifications in the isolation protocol such as adding other media or using different growth conditions.

Gross examination of clinical specimens is typically of limited value, except when nodules are present on hairs. *Piedraia hortae* forms black nodules that are hard, variable in size, and firmly attached to the hair shaft. If one draws their fingers along the hair shaft, the nodules

Figure 1.1 Tinea corporis. The edge of the skin is scraped with a #15 scalpel blade.

Figure 1.2 *Malassezia furfur (Pityrosporum)* periodic acid–Schiff (PAS) stain demonstrating yeasts and hyphae in skin scales.

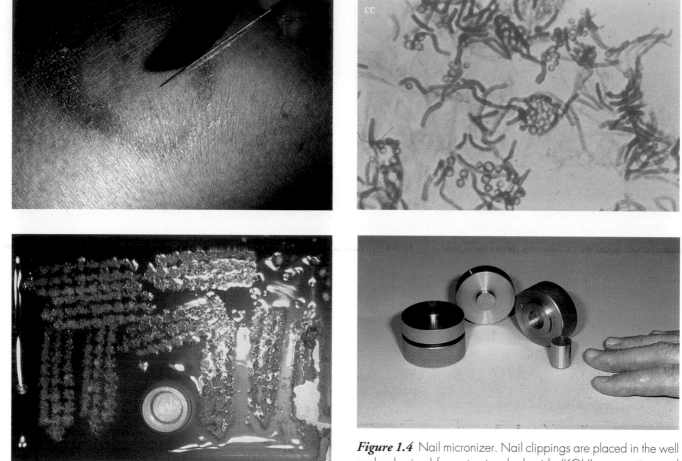

Figure 1.4 Nail micronizer. Nail clippings are placed in the well and pulverized for potassium hydroxide (KOH) preparation and culture.

Figure 1.3 Tinea capitis. A toothbrush was used to collect infected debris from the scalp. The brush was touched on the surface of the medium containing rapid sprouting medium (RSM).

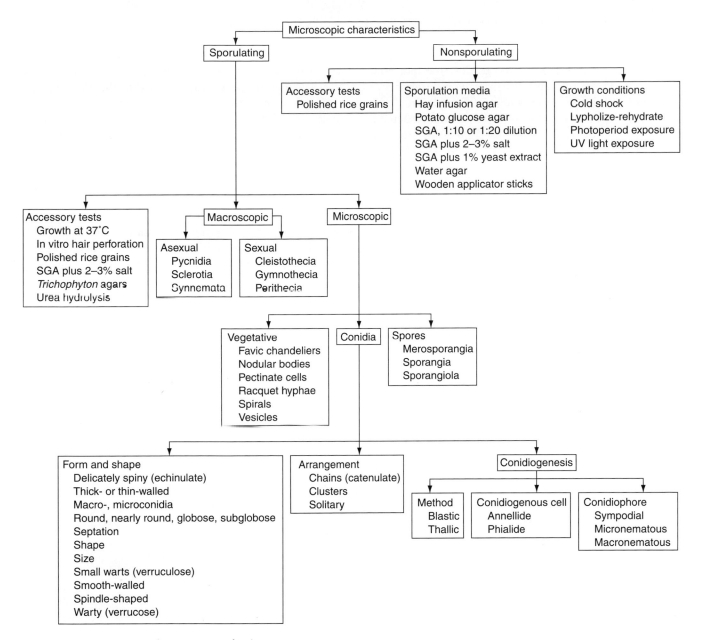

Figure 1.5 Microscopic characteristics of colonies.

will not become dislodged. In contrast, a nodule formed by *Trichosporon beigelii* will easily become dislodged as the hair shaft passes through the fingers. *Black* and *white piedra* are the names used to describe hair colonization by these two fungi, respectively. Microscopically, the nodules of *P. hortae* contain cylindric, nonseptate, hyaline ascospores having ends that taper into narrow filaments. The nodules of *T. beigelii* are composed of hyphae that fragment into arthroconidia.

To visualize fungal elements in hair, nail, and skin, a solution of 10 to 20% potassium hydroxide (KOH) is used to clear the clinical material. Fungi are temporarily resistant to the action of the KOH because they have ridged cell walls containing chitin. Within a few days, however, fungi will decompose too. Hence, KOH preparations are not permanent. The addition of chlorazol E or Parker's ink (Fig. 1.1) to KOH (Fig. 1.6) or calcofluor white to KOH will stain the fungal elements and render them more visible. Calcofluor white requires the use of a fluorescent microscope because it is a nonspecific fluorescent dye that attaches to chitin and cellulose. For better penetration into nail tissue, dimethyl sulfoxide (DMSO) can be carefully added to the KOH.

Hyphae, pseudohyphae, and yeast cells are easily seen, especially if a phase-contrast microscope is used in conjunction with a bright field optics. Hairs present more of a challenge. Immediately examine hairs when they are first placed in a mounting medium such as KOH. Fungi such as *Trichophyton schoenleinii* form hyphae that decompose within the hair shaft, resulting in channels. Air bubbles can be seen racing down the hair shaft as the mounting medium is pulled by capillary action down the hair shaft. This type of hair invasion during the natural infection is a form of endothrix invasion (Fig. 1.7). In most instances of endothrix invasion, the hyphae within the hair shaft fragment into arthroconidia.

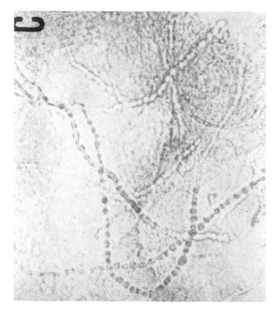

Figure 1.6 A KOH preparation. Note long, branching hyphae.

Figure 1.7 Infected hair—endothrix invasion.

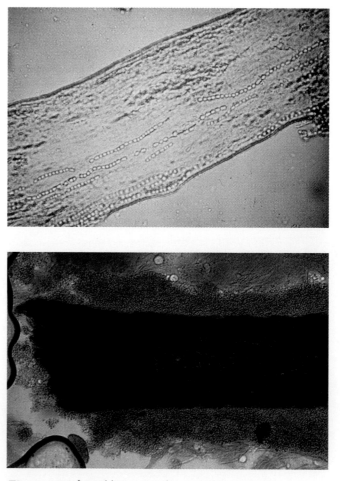

Figure 1.8 Infected hair—ectothrix invasion.

The second type of hair invasion is ectothrix (Fig. 1.8). In this case, the fungus grows within the hair and on its surface. The hyphae fragment into arthroconidia, resulting in conidia being present in and around the hair. In ectothrix invasion, the cuticle of the hair is destroyed; this does not occur in endothrix invasion.

ISOLATION OF ETIOLOGIC AGENTS

Isolation of the etiologic agent is important. With the exception of *M. furfur* and *P. hortae,* the fungi must be cultured before they can be accurately identified. The identified fungi can be correlated with the observations of the fungal elements in the clinical specimens, guide therapy options, provide epidemiologic data, and can be used for in vitro antifungal susceptibility testing.

Media with and without 0.04% cycloheximide should always be used for primary isolation because many of the etiologic agents of the dermatomycosis, such as *Scopulariopsis brevicaulis,* are sensitive to cycloheximide. Dermatophytes are not sensitive to this antifungal agent, hence its popularity for recovering dermatophytes and eliminating fungi that were once thought only to be contaminants. Mycosel and mycobiotic agars contain cycloheximide as well as 0.005% chloramphenicol to inhibit bacterial growth. Sabouraud's dextrose agar (SGA), mold inhibitory agar, SGA plus gentamicin, and dermatophyte test medium (DTM) are also used for primary isolation. DTM is not a good primary isolation medium except for specimens heavily contaminated with fungi and bacteria that will activate the phenol red indicator. Fungi on DTM do not exhibit the typical colonial morphology, color, or microscopic characteristics that are necessary for the accurate identification of dermatophytes.

Isolation media can be placed in either Petri dishes, bottles, or test tubes. Petri dishes offer increased surface area for the specimens and are easy to work with. Dehydration can be reduced by wrapping oxygen permeable tape around the edge of the dish. If bottles or test tubes are used, their caps must be kept loose to ensure gas exchange. The isolation media are incubated at 25 to 30°C for approximately 14 days. Fungi such as *Trichophyton concentricum* and *T. schoenleinii* may require 4 weeks of incubation.

IDENTIFICATION

Identification of the isolated fungi provides valuable information. First, it clarifies which fungus or fungi are in-

volved. This information has epidemiologic importance in determining the distribution and frequency of the different dermatophyte species. The name of the fungus serves as a literature entry point to determine the experience of others in treating similar cases. If unusual fungi are isolated, the repeated isolation of the same species may be valuable information for differential diagnosis.

Yeasts are identified using a combination of physiologic and morphologic criteria. When species like *C. albicans* are involved, rapid tests, such as germ-tube production, are used for identification. Other yeasts require physiologic data for their accurate identification.

Molds are identified (Figs. 1.9 to 1.19) based on their gross colonial characteristics and microscopic structure. For dermatophytes, SGA is used to study the colonial characteristics necessary for their identification. Some individuals supplement this system with 1% yeast extract to induce faster growth, more conidia, and better pigment production. The addition of 2 to 3% sodium chloride to the medium stimulates macroconidium production in species like *Trichophyton mentagrophytes* and retards pleomorphic colony development in other species such as *Epidermophyton floccosum*

The production of conidia can be enhanced by using a 1:10 or 1:20 dilution of SGA or other media such as potato glucose agar, corn meal agar, V-8 juice agar, hay infusion agar, or 2% water agar. Numerous other substrates and various environmental manipulations can be used to stimulate the production of conidia or macroscopic structures like pycnidia.

Dermatophyte colonies are distinctive for each of the species. At times, supplemental tests such as the following will be necessary: *Trichophyton* agars, polished rice grains to distinguish *Microsporum audouinii* and *Microsporum canis,* urea hydrolysis, or the in vitro perforation of hair to separate *T. mentagrophytes* and *Trichophyton rubrum* (Fig. 1.19), growth at 37°C to distinguish *T. mentagrophytes* from *Trichophyton terrestre,* and the use of enriched media incubated at 37°C to develop chlamydoconidia by *Trichophyton verrucosum.*

Microscopic observations need to be made with care. They can be valuable in determining the purity of the isolate, especially if the colonial characteristics suggest that more than one organism is present: mold-dermatophyte, dermatophyte-dermatophyte, mold-mold, or a yeast or bacterium with each of these combinations. A pure culture is necessary for accurate identification. Mixed infections of two or more fungi contributing to the infection at the same time are not uncommon.

Figure 1.9 (A–C) *Trichophyton rubrum.* The culture is white, fluffy to granular. A nondiffusing red pigment under the thallus is characteristic. Microconidia are peg-shaped, uniform in size, and diagnostic. Occasionally thin-walled, pencil-shaped macroconidia are produced.

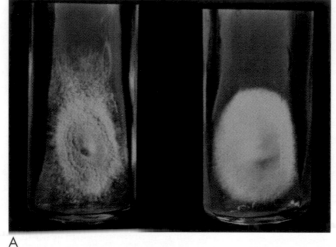

A

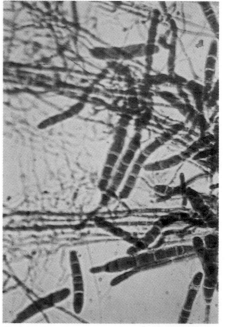

B

C

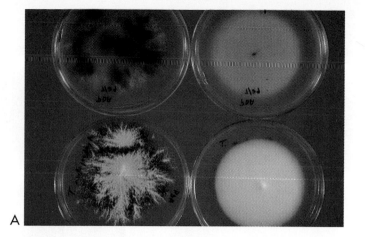

Figure 1.10 (A&B) *Trichophyton mentagrophytes.* The texture of the colony is woolly or silky white (var. *interdigitalis*) to powdery (var. *mentagrophytes*). The surface is white to creamy in color. Microconidia are spherical in grape-like clusters. In downy strains, clavate-shaped conidia are seen. Some strains show spiral hyphal cells. The macroconidia have thin walls like the macroconidia of *Trichophyton rubrum*.

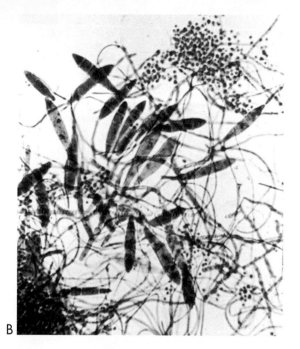

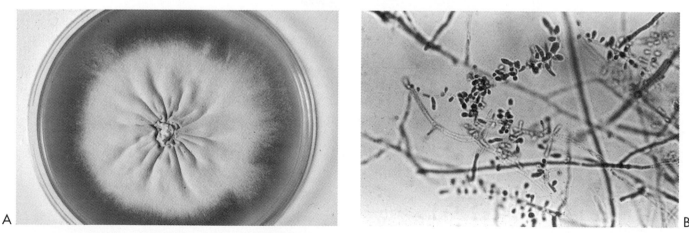

Figure 1.11 (A&B) *Trichophyton tonsurans.* On primary isolation, the colony is powdery milk-yellow tinged. The colony develops into a folded thallus with a suede-like surface. Growth is enhanced by the addition of thiamine. The microconidia of *T. tonsurans* are variable in size and shape. They may be clavate or spherical, and several of these microconidia may enlarge, becoming balloon-shaped.

Figure 1.12 (A–C) *Trichophyton verrucosum*. The colony is slightly folded, heaped, glabrous, and gray-white. The growth is enhanced by a temperature of 37°C. At 37°C, the fungus grows as a chain of chlamydoconidia (a reliable test). At room temperature, distorted hyphae suggesting antler-branching can be seen. "Rat-tail" macroconidia are characteristic when present.

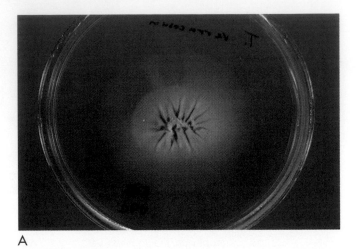

A

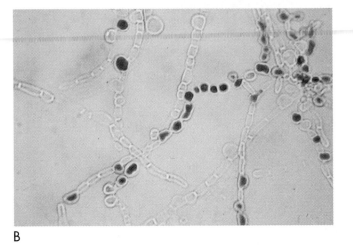

B

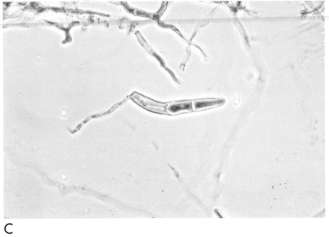

C

Figure 1.13 (A&B) *Trichophyton schoenleinii.* A slow-growing glabrous (waxy) or suede-like off-white colony. Conidia are not seen. The hyphae form antler-like structures.

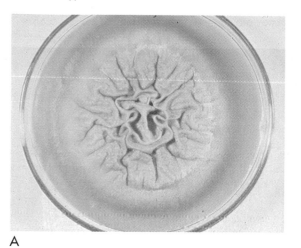

A

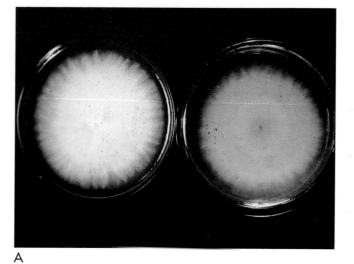

A

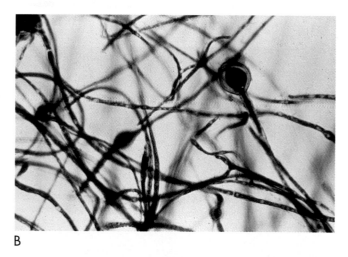

B

B

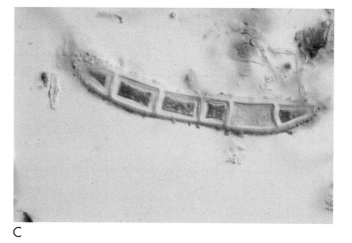

C

Figure 1.14 *Microsporum violaceum.* A very slow-growing, glabrous (waxy) colony that is deep violet in color. Distorted hyphae and lack of conidia are typical. (A) Primary isolate. (B) Subculture (note loss of deep violet color).

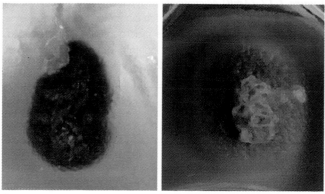

A   B

Figure 1.15 (A–C) *Microsporum audouinii.* The colony is woolly with radiating edges. The color is white or gray to rust or buff. The back of the colony is fresh pink. Generally very few to no microdia are present. Thick-walled terminal or intercalary chlamydoconidia are characteristic. Macroconidia, if present, are irregular in shape, elongated, thick-walled, and echinulate.

SUGGESTED READING

Aly R: Culture media for growing dermatophytes. J Am Acad Dermatol 31:5107, 1994

Haley LD, Calloway CS: Laboratory Methods in Medical Mycology. 4th Ed. HEW Publication No. (CDC) 78-8361. Centers for Disease Control, Atlanta, 1978

McGinnis MR: Laboratory Handbook of Medical Mycology. Academic Press, New York, 1980

Rippon JW: Medical Mycology: The Pathogenic Fungi and the Pathogenic Actinomycetes. 3rd Ed. WB Saunders, New York, 1988

Weitzman I, Kane J, Summerbell RC: *Trichophyton, Microsporum, Epidermophyton* and agents of superficial mycoses. p. 791. In Murray PR et al (eds): Manual of Clinical Microbiology. 6th Ed. American Society for Microbiology, Washington, DC, 1995

CHAPTER 2

Superficial Mycoses and Dermatophytoses

Raza Aly

Aditya K. Gupta

SUMMARY

Etiology   There are a large number of fungi that cause infections of the skin, scalp, and nails

Clinical Features   Tinea nigra, black piedra, white piedra, tinea capitis, tinea barbae, tinea faciei, tinea corporis, tinea cruris, tinea pedis, onychomycosis

Pathology   Biopsy may be indicated in some clinical conditions

Diagnosis   Clinical presentation, microscopic examination of potassium hydroxide–treated skin scrapings, and culture

Treatment   Antifungal therapies

Differential Diagnosis   Tinea nigra (malignant melanoma, lentigo, chemical stains, junctional nevi); black piedra (nits, trichosporosis of the scalp, trichomycosis); white piedra (trichomycosis axillaris); tinea capitis (seborrheic dermatitis, psoriasis, atopic dermatitis, pediculosis capitis); tinea barbae (bacterial folliculitis, carbuncle, candidal dermatitis, herpes simplex or zoster, actinomycosis, perioral dermatitis, acneiform dermatitis, pseudofolliculitis, contact dermatitis, iododerma or bromoderma); tinea faciei (eczema, psoriasis, seborrheic dermatitis, impetigo, bowenoid actinic dermatitis, polymorphous light eruption, discoid lupus erythematosus, acne rosacea, benign lymphocytic infiltrate); tinea corporis (erythema annulare centrifugum, granuloma annulare, psoriasis, seborrheic dermatitis, nummular eczema, pityriasis rosea, erythema multiforme, erythrasma, impetigo, lichen planus, secondary syphilis); tinea cruris (intertrigo, candidiasis, erythrasma, psoriasis, atopic dermatitis, mycosis fungoides, pityriasis versicolor, flexural Darier's disease, Hailey-Hailey disease, contact or irritant dermatitis); tinea pedis (toe cleft impetigo, contact dermatitis, pustular psoriasis, interdigital intertrigo, idiopathic hyperkeratosis, erysipelas, pitted keratolysis, fixed drug eruption); onychomycosis (infections due to nondermatophytic fungi, psoriasis, lichen planus, trauma, onychogryphosis)

SUPERFICIAL MYCOSES

Tinea Nigra

Etiology   Tinea nigra is most common in tropical and subtropical climates and has been reported in North and South America, Asia, and Africa. The etiologic agent *Phaeoannellomyces werneckii* (*Cladosporium werneckii*, *Exophiala werneckii*) is a demataceous fungus. It is isolated from soil, beach sand, and salted freshwater fish. Predisposing factors to infection are not known.

Clinical Features   Tinea nigra is a superficial infection of the stratum corneum (Table 2.1) characterized by brown to black nonscaly macules with pronounced delineated margins. Lesions typically favor the palm but may occur on soles or other surfaces of the skin as well. The lesion starts as a light brown macule that spreads centrifugally (Fig. 2.1).

Table 2.1 Fungi Infecting Only the Superficial Layers of Hair and Stratum Corneum

MICROORGANISM	DISEASE
Phaeoannellomyces werneckii (*Cladosporium werneckii*, *Exophiala werneckii*)	Tinea nigra
Piedraia hortae	Black piedra
Trichosporon beigelii	White piedra
Malassezia furfur (*Pityrosporum* species)	Pityriasis (tinea) versicolor

Figure 2.2 *Phaeoannellomyces werneckii.* Note dark, pigmented, septate hyphae.

Figure 2.1 Tinea nigra. A typical lesion on the palmar surface, a brown-black nonscaly macule.

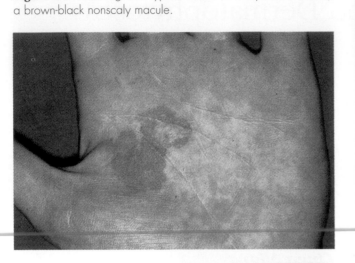

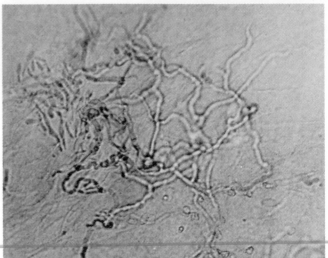

Figure 2.3 *Phaeoannello-myces werneckii.* A moist, black-colored colony.

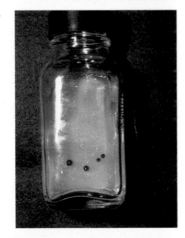

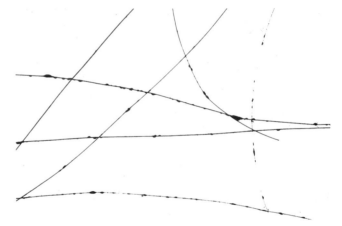

Figure 2.4 Black piedra. Note small black nodules along the lesion.

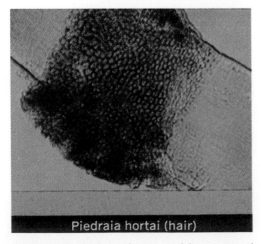
Piedraia hortai (hair)

Figure 2.5 Black piedra. A nodule examined under the light microscope.

Pathology There is little or no host reaction to the infection. Biopsy shows proliferation of dermataceous hyphae and elongated yeast cells in the upper layers of the stratum corneum. Rarely, some parakeratosis and a small amount of perivascular lymphocytic filtrate may be seen.

Diagnosis Diagnosis is made on the typical clinical presentation and by microscopic examination of potassium hydroxide (KOH)–treated skin scrapings taken from a pigmented lesion. Observation at low magnification reveals dark, branched, septate hyphae and budding cells (Fig. 2.2). Microscopy of cultured growth demonstrates a dermataceous fungus with characteristic one- or two-celled conidia, *P. werneckii,* which when cultured forms a dark-colored colony (Fig. 2.3).

Treatment The lesion responds to topical ketoconazole and other azole creams. Whitfield's ointment will clear the condition readily. Topical thiabendazole has been used successfully.[2]

Prognosis If untreated, the lesions may be persistent. However, spontaneous resolution is common.

Differential Diagnosis Tinea nigra should be differentiated from malignant melanoma, lentigo, chemical stains, and junctional nevi.

Black Piedra

Etiology Black piedra is an infection of the skin by *Piedraia hortae* characterized by the presence of small black nodules along the hair shaft. The disease is found in the western hemisphere, the tropics, and Indonesia.

Clinical Features Nodules of black piedra are gritty, hard, brown to black encrustations of the hair shaft (Figs. 2.4 and 2.5). The disease is only of cosmetic concern, as the patient experiences no discomfort or physical reaction. The scalp itself is not involved.

Pathology The periphery of the mature nodule is composed of elongated hyphal strands, whereas fungal cells in the central area are cemented together to form a pseudoparenchymatous mass that resembles organized tissue. Mature nodules can be crushed to reveal oval asci containing two to eight fusiform ascospores.

Diagnosis Microscopic examination of nodules in KOH preparation shows pigmented hyphae cemented together in a mass asci and ascospores. *P. hortae* is a dermataceous fungus.

Treatment The best and most simple treatment is cutting off the infected hair. The disease responds to oral terbinafine.[3]

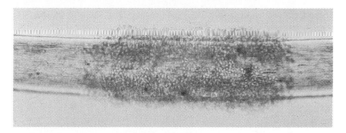

Figure 2.6 White piedra. Soft nodules around the hair.

Differential Diagnosis The disease must be distinguished from nits, trichosporosis of the scalp, and trichomycosis. The latter two infections may be stripped from the hair with relative ease.

White Piedra

Etiology White piedra is induced by *Trichosporon beigelii.* This microorganism grows around the hair shaft, forming a soft sleeve of intertwined hyphae that breaks into yeast-like arthroconidia.

Clinical Features The disease is characterized by soft, easily detached, white to brown granules along the hair shaft. The infection is more common in the bearded regions, the axilla, and the groin. The scalp is less frequently involved. It has been reported that the carrier rate of *T. beigelii* in the anal area is higher in homosexual men.[4]

The infection starts beneath the cuticle. The microorganism grows inward and through the shaft, thus producing nodules. Hair thereby becomes weakened and brittle and is often broken. Several nodules may merge to form an extensive mass around the hair shaft. Piedra does not fluoresce under ultraviolet light (Figs. 2.6).

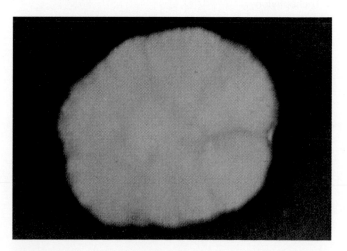

Figure 2.7 Creamy-white colonies of *Trichosporon beigelii.*

Diagnosis The granules in white piedra are softer and more easily detached from hair than black piedra. The microorganism grows both within the hair shaft and on the surface. KOH preparations reveal hyaline hyphal elements, arthroconidia, and blastoconidia. Growth on Sabouraud's agar is rapid (4 to 5 days); the colonies are creamy white in color (Fig. 2.7).

Treatment Shaving of affected hair and topical amphotericin B are recommended. Topical imidazoles are also used.

Differential Diagnosis Trichomycosis axillaris should be distinguished from white piedra. They can be differentiated by culture and direct microscopy.

DERMATOPHYTOSES

Tinea Capitis

Etiology There are three species of dermatophytes that are pathogenic in humans: *Trichophyton, Microsporum,* and *Epidermophyton,* with only the first two causing tinea capitis. The organisms that do not exhibit hair invasion include *Trichophyton concentricum, Epidermophyton floccosum,* and *Microsporum persicolor.* In the United States, the majority of tinea capitis is due to *Trichophyton tonsurans* and *Microsporum canis* infection.[5] The three patterns of hair invasion that cause tinea capitis are ectothrix, endothrix, and favus (Table 2.2). In

Table 2.2 Organisms that Cause Tinea Capitis

SPECIES	ECTOTHRIX ENDOTHRIX FAVUS	FLUORESCENT (F) NONFLUORESCENT (NF)	SIZE OF CONIDIA OR SPORE SMALL: 2–3 μm LARGE: 5–8 μm	ANTHROPOPHILIC (A) ZOOPHILIC (Z) GEOPHILIC (G)	GEOGRAPHIC DISTRIBUTION
Microsporum					
M. audouinii	Ecto	F	Small	A	Worldwide
M. canis	Ecto	F	Small	Z	Worldwide
M. distortum	Ecto	F	Small	Z	Australia
M. ferrugineum	Ecto	F	Small	A	Asia, Africa
M. equinum	Ecto	F	Small	Z	Worldwide
M. gypseum	Ecto/Favus	NF, occasionally F	Large	G	Worldwide
M. nanum	Ecto	NF	Large	Z/G	Worldwide
M. fulvum	Ecto	NF	Large	G	South America
M. vanbreuseghemii	Ecto	NF	Large	G/Z	Africa, India
M. gallinae	Ecto	NF	Large	Z	Worldwide
Trichophyton					
T. verrucosum	Ecto	NF	Large	Z	Worldwide
T. mentagrophytes	Ecto	NF	Large	Z/A	Worldwide
T. megninii	Ecto	NF	Large	A	Europe
T. rubrum	Ecto/rarely Endo	NF	Large	A	Worldwide
T. tonsurans	Endo	NF	Large	A	Worldwide
T. violaceum	Endo/Favus	NF	Large	A	Worldwide
T. soudanense	Endo	NF	Large	A	Africa
T. yaoundei	Endo	NF	Large	A	Africa
T. gourvilii	Endo	NF	Large	A	Africa
T. schoenleinii	Favus	F	No spores	A	Europe

general, *Microsporum* ectothrix infection caused by small-sized conidia or spores (2 to 3 μm in diameter) gives fluorescent tinea capitis, whereas that associated with large-sized conidia (5 to 8 μm in diameter) results in nonfluorescent disease. Ectothrix or endothrix infection caused by *Trichophyton* species gives nonfluorescent tinea capitis. In humans, favus infection is associated with *Trichophyton schoenleinii*. The clinical appearance of the tinea capitis is generally dependent on the immune response of the host and not the etiologic agent. Tinea capitis is usually seen in children between the ages of 4 and 14 years. Infections in adults are uncommon and when they occur are usually due to *Trichophyton* species. *Microsporum* infections in children occur more commonly in males. In contrast, *T. tonsurans* in children affects males and females almost equally. African-Americans and Hispanics may have a higher prevalence of tinea capitis due to *T. tonsurans*; however, in whites, *M. canis* infection may be more common. In some instances, the transmission of tinea capitis is favored by overcrowding and poor hygiene. Factors that favor the spread of infection include the fact that spores with the potential to cause tinea capitis have been cultured from inanimate objects that the infected subject may have come in contact with, for example, combs, hairbrushes, caps, helmets, pillows, and so on. Furthermore, hair shed off the scalp from a subject with tinea capitis may remain infective for over a year.[6] The asymptomatic carrier state may play a role in the persistence of tinea capitis.[7]

The organisms that produce tinea capitis can be broadly classified according to the host preference (anthropophilic, zoophilic, or geophilic) and the site of infection in relation to the hair shaft (endothrix [infection within the hair] or ectothrix [infection just under hair cuticle]).

The fungi that cause tinea capitis vary from country to country (Table 2.2). Also over time the species that cause tinea capitis may change in a given area. In the United States, there has been an increase in tinea capitis due to *T. tonsurans*. Likewise, in Europe, *M. canis* has become more prevalent.

Clinical Features The noninflammatory type of tinea capitis is often caused by *Microsporum audouinii, M. canis, Microsporum ferrugineum,* and *T. tonsurans*. Initially, a small erythematous papule may be present. It spreads outward, producing one or more "gray" patches that exhibit minimal inflammation (Fig. 2.8). The term *gray* refers to coating of arthrospores on the scalp surface. Hair often break off just above the level of the scalp. The clinical presentation varies from hair loss with scaling of the involved area to areas of minimal scale that resemble seborrheic dermatitis.

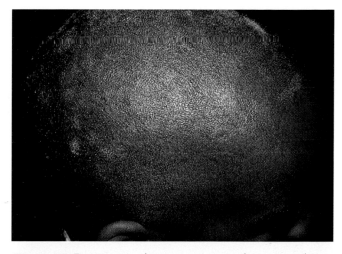

Figure 2.8 Tinea capitis showing a gray patch variety with minimal inflammation. (Courtesy of Dr. Ilona Frieden.)

In the inflammatory type of tinea capitis, the hallmark is the presence of significantly more inflammation. Infections are typically caused by zoophilic species (e.g., *M. canis*) or geophilic organisms (e.g., *M. gypseum*). A spectrum of presentations may be observed, varying from a pustular folliculitis or multiple follicular abscesses to a kerion. In a kerion, the organism is usually a zoophilic species, although less frequently geophilic and anthropophilic organisms may be implicated (Fig. 2.9). The lesion may be single or sometimes multiple, consisting of a painful, inflammatory, boggy mass with broken hair follicles. There may be several areas that are discharging pus, sometimes with sinus formation. The kerion may progress to exhibit complete loss of hair in the involved area, sometimes resulting in scarring alopecia. The inflammatory cutaneous response can be accompanied by symptoms of pyrexia, pain, pruritus, and cervical and regional lymphadenopathy. A kerion may be the manifestation of a hypersensitivity reaction, and occasionally an id reaction may be observed at other sites. A concomitant bacterial infection should be excluded.

Black dot tinea capitis is due to endothrix organisms such as *T. tonsurans* and *T. violaceum*. The hair is brittle and breaks off at the scalp surface, leaving behind a black dot (Fig. 2.10). The clinical presentation may vary from minimal inflammation and diffuse scaling with little evidence of alopecia with black dot infection and inflammatory changes that range from a pustular folliculitis to a kerion. In some instances, scarring and permanent alopecia may develop.

In the favus variety of tinea capitis, dermatophytes that have been implicated are *T. schoenleinii* and less frequently *T. violaceum* and *M. gypseum*. The condition may be familial. It is endemic in areas such as the Mid-

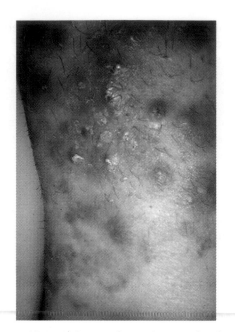

Figure 2.18 Majocchi's granuloma. Lesions developed on a young female patient.

ple with erythema, inflammatory perifollicular nodules, or pustules. Lesions may develop on the legs of women probably as a consequence of inoculation of fungal organisms when shaving the legs. In such instances, *T. rubrum* may be cultured. Nodular granulomatous changes may also be seen at other anatomic sites. Infrequently, patients may experience subcutaneous and systemic spread of fungal organisms with deep subcutaneous nodules, abscesses, and sinus formation. In rare instances, there may be lymph node involvement and systemic spread.

Changes similar to favus in the scalp may be observed when *T. schoenleinii* infects glabrous skin. Tinea corporis may occasionally be of the bullous variety. Possible infecting organisms include *T. rubrum*. Tinea imbricata (tokelau) is caused by the anthropophilic dermatophyte *T. concentricum*. Multiple, concentric, annular rings are present.

Pathology   When the infection is due to *Trichophyton* and *Microsporum* species, hyphae may be observed in the horny layers of the stratum corneum. Generally there is no penetration of the hair follicles except with *T. rubrum* and *T. verrucosum*. In this instance, a perifolliculitis is present with hyphae in the dermal infiltrate. When fungi cannot be demonstrated, the histopathology of tinea of the glabrous skin (tinea corporis, tinea cruris, tinea faciei) is similar to acute, subacute, or chronic dermatitis depending on the degree of inflammatory response.

Diagnosis   Skin scrapings should be obtained from the actively advancing margin of the lesion and the KoH preparation examined under light microscopy. A culture helps in the definitive isolation of the causative organism. When granulomatous lesions are present, it may be necessary to perform a biopsy. In bullous lesions, the roof of the blister may give the best yield of fungal organisms.

Treatment   Tinea corporis is normally treated by topical agents such as the imidazoles (e.g., miconazole, clotrimazole, or ketoconazole), the allylamines (terbinafine, naftifine, or butenafine), tolnaftate, or ciclopirox olamine. When the eruption involves a large surface area, or if there is a poor response to topical agents, then oral therapy should be considered. Possible choices include griseofulvin, ketoconazole, terbinafine, or fluconazole. The newer antifungal agents are effective and are being used increasingly more frequently than the traditional agents griseofulvin and ketoconazole. When the fungal infection involves hair follicles, dermal tissues, or deeper tissues, then oral antifungal therapy should be regarded as first-line therapy.

Differential Diagnosis   When lesions are annular, other conditions to consider are erythema annulare centrifugum and granuloma annulare. When the eruption is more red and scaly, the differential diagnosis includes psoriasis (Fig. 2.19), seborrheic dermatitis (Fig. 2.20), nummular eczema, pityriasis rosea (Fig. 2.21), erythema multiforme (Fig. 2.22), erythrasma, impetigo, lichen planus (Fig. 2.23) and secondary syphilis. When the fungal infection involves the dermis and deeper tissues, the differential diagnosis includes bacterial infections and mycoses involving the dermis and subcutaneous tissue.

Tinea Cruris

Etiology   The most common organisms are *T. rubrum, E. floccosum,* and *T. mentagrophytes*. It should be noted that tinea cruris is the only dermatophyte where *E. floccosum* may be prominent as an etiologic agent. Tinea cruris is found more frequently in males. Factors that facilitate infection are warm, humid weather; use of occlusive clothing for long periods of time, especially if it is wet or humid; and the use of articles of personal hygiene or clothing infected with the organism implicated in tinea cruris, for example, towels, bedsheets, or certain items of sportswear. Obesity, diabetes mellitus, and poor personal hygiene may also increase the probability of developing tinea cruris. The presence of tinea infection at other anatomic sites, for example, tinea pedis, may serve as a reservoir of infection. Close physical contact with a person with tinea cruris does not necessarily

Figure 2.19 Psoriasis.

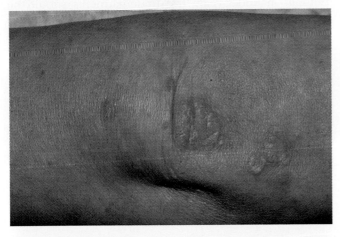

Figure 2.20 Seborrheic dermatitis.

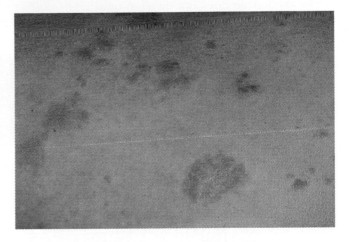

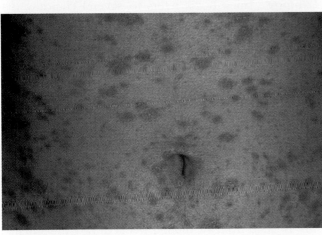

Figure 2.21 Pityriasis rosea.

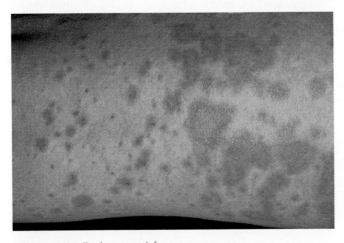

Figure 2.22 Erythema multiforme.

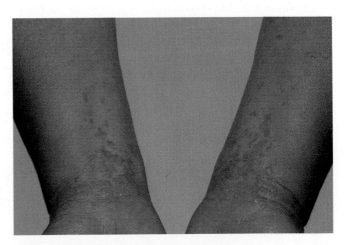

Figure 2.23 Lichen planus.

result in infection. This has been observed in partners where the female does not develop tinea cruris despite the presence of disease in the male partner.

Clinical Features   Pruritus may be present. The eruption may be symmetric or asymmetric, unilateral or bilateral (Fig. 2.24). The clinical presentation may provide a clue to the etiologic agent; for example, with *E. floccosum* infection, there may be an active, inflammatory eruption with papules or vesicles at the border and central clearing. Infections caused by *T. rubrum* are more likely to be chronic and involve a wider area of the perineum. With *Candida* species, lesions may be present on the scrotum or penis. In adults, it is not as common to see satellite pustules associated with *Candida* species infection, a presentation often seen in children (Fig. 2.25).

Pathology   The histopathologic findings are similar to those seen in tinea corporis.

Diagnosis   The clinical suspicion is confirmed by obtaining skin scrapings from the active border followed by examination under a light microscope and seeding a culture.

Treatment   For the active condition, topical antifungal therapy is generally sufficient. When the tinea cruris is widespread or recalcitrant, oral antifungal agents such as itraconazole, terbinafine, or griseofulvin may need to be considered. Of these antifungal agents, itraconazole appears to have the widest spectrum of action.

Attention should be paid to the appropriate treatment of any reservoir for infection, for example, tinea pedis. The history provided by the patient will help identify predisposing factors for the tinea cruris, and appropriate measures should be undertaken to reduce the risk of reinfection. This may involve washing the affected area regularly and ensuring that it is completely dry before putting on underwear. The undergarments should be relatively loose and made of appropriate material. The use of absorbent powders may be beneficial. The individual should refrain from sharing items of infected clothing that may aid in the spread of the infection.

Differential Diagnosis   The differential diagnosis includes intertrigo, candidiasis (Fig. 2.26), erythrasma (Figs. 2.27, 2.28), psoriasis, atopic dermatitis, mycosis fungoides, pityriasis versicolor, flexural Darier's disease, Hailey-Hailey disease, and contact or irritant dermatitis.

Tinea Pedis

Etiology   Tinea pedis refers to several clinically distinct fungal infections of the foot. Dermatophytes are primarily involved; however, nondermatophytes—molds and yeasts—can also produce disease clinically indistinguishable from tinea pedis. The common etiologic agents of tinea pedis are listed in Table 2.3.

Foot infection is the most common form of superficial fungal infection, involving up to 70% of the population.[14] Tinea pedis occurs more often in adult men than in women and children. Tinea pedis is more common among people who frequent swimming pools or use community washing facilities, such as found in army camps, boarding schools, and prisons. The high incidence of *T. rubrum, T. mentagrophytes,* and *E. floccosum* isolated from swimming pools during the summer months testifies to the effective spread of tinea pedis. Tinea pedis occurs mainly among people who wear enclosed shoes and sneakers, which probably contribute to an increasing frequency. The single most important factor that regulates the incidence, prevalence, and severity of tinea pedis is occlusion.[15]

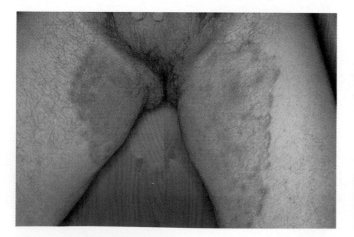

Figure 2.24 Tinea cruris. Extension of lesion on the thigh area.

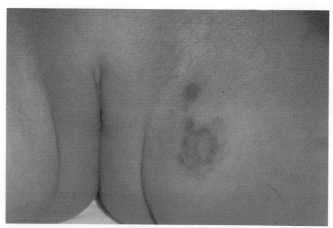

Figure 2.25 Tinea cruris. A rare infection in an infant.

Figure 2.26 Vulvovaginitis involving the crural area.

Figure 2.27 Erythrasma of the groin caused by *Corynebacterium minutissimum*.

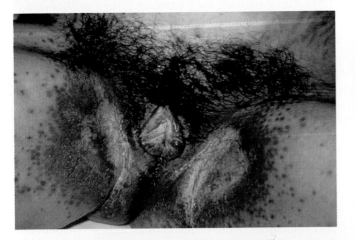

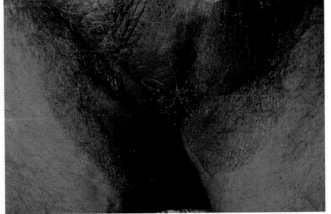

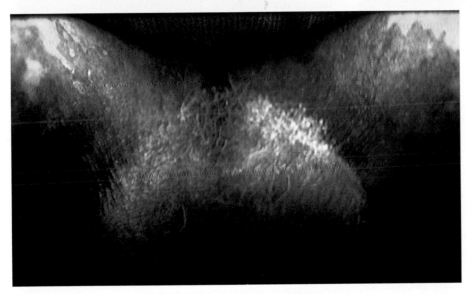

Figure 2.28 Erythrasma that fluoresces red under Wood's light.

Table 2.3 Causative Agents of Tinea Pedis

PATTERN	CAUSITIVE ORGANISM
Interdigital type	*Trichophyton mentagrophytes*
	Trichophyton rubrum
	Epidermophyton floccosum
	Candida albicans
	Scytalidium dimidiatum
	Scytalidium hyalinum
Moccasin type	*T. rubrum*
	T. mentagrophytes
	E. floccosum
	S. dimidiatum
	S. hyalinum
Vesiculobullous type	*T. mentagrophytes*
Ulcerative type	*T. rubrum*
	T. mentagrophytes
	E. floccosum
	Candida albicans[a]
	Staphylococcus aureus[a]

[a] Present as a copathogen or colonizer.

Clinical Features The three major clinical types of tinea pedis are the interdigital type, the moccasin or chronic hyperkeratotic type, and the highly inflammatory vesiculobullous type (Table 2.3). A fourth clinical type, ulcerative tinea pedis, the rarest of tinea pedis, is encountered mainly in immunocompromised patients.

Interdigital Tinea Pedis Interdigital tinea pedis is the most common type. The areas between the fourth and fifth toes and the third and fourth toes are most often involved. The clinical spectrum ranges from relatively asymptomatic mild scaling to exudative, macerated, and malodorous conditions (Figs. 2.29 to 2.31).

In macerated, malodorous lesions, there is an overgrowth of the resident flora between the toes. Secondary infection due to bacteria, typically *Staphylococcus aureus* and *Pseudomonas* species, may further complicate the picture. The recovery of dermatophytes from macerated, exudative interspaces is low. Uncomplicated dry, scaly-type tinea pedis is referred to as dermatophytosis simplex, while the macerated, complicated type is called dermatophytosis complex.[16]

Plantar, Moccasin-Type Tinea Pedis Plantar, moccasin-type tinea pedis is characterized by a dull erythema, dryness, subtly scaling, and hyperkeratosis affecting the entire plantar skin of the feet in sandal or moccasin

distribution (Fig. 2.32). At times, one hand will be similarly involved with this diffuse scaling condition (Fig. 2.33). These patients have a defect in their cell-mediated immunity, being unable to mount a delayed-type hypersensitivity response, which is the host mechanism by which fungi are eliminated. Patients with moccasin-type tinea pedis often have toenail infections (Fig. 2.34). This moccasin type of infection is recalcitrant to ordinary treatments. Resistance could be related to the fact that the stratum corneum of the plantar surface is too thick for drugs to penetrate. For successful treatment of this type of tinea pedis, any toenail infection should also be dealt with. *T. rubrum* is frequently associated with moccasin tinea pedis.

Vesiculobullous Tinea Pedis Vesiculobullous lesions are often seen on the instep or mid anterior plantar surface or dorsal surface. The eruptions occur typically with vesicles and bullae in clusters (Figs. 2.35 to 2.37). This form is often responsible for the production of the id reaction on the hand. During primary infection, a brisk T-cell immune response develops, which produces an allergic response to the fungus. At times the inflammatory response is so acute that cellulitis, lymphangitis, and adenopathy occur and are incapacitating. The vesicular form of the tinea pedis is most often caused by *T. mentagrophytes*.

Ulcerative Tinea Pedis Ulcerative tinea pedis is usually associated with immunocompromised patients. The disease is complicated by secondary bacterial infection (Fig. 2.38).

Nondermatophytes and Tinea Pedis Several nondermatophytes have been implicated in foot and nail infections, but their etiology is often difficult to establish. *Scytalidium dimidiatum* (*Hendersonula toruloidea*) and *Scytalidium hyalinum* have been reported as agents of recalcitrant foot and nail infections[17,18] (Figs. 2.39 and 2.40). *S. dimidiatum* does not respond to griseofulvin, imidazoles, or terbinafine.

Pathology With the exception of fungal elements among the keratinous layers, no specific changes are seen. An acute, subacute, or chronic dermatitis may be present.

Diagnosis The diagnosis of tinea pedis is confirmed by direct microscopic examination of infected scales in KOH slide mount. The infected scales should be removed from the periphery of the lesions. If bullae are present, these are clipped, examined, and cultured. Any antifungal or topical creams must be removed before culturing material. Even if the KOH preparation is nega-

Text continued on page 32

Figure 2.29 Interdigital tinea pedis. Mild scaly type.

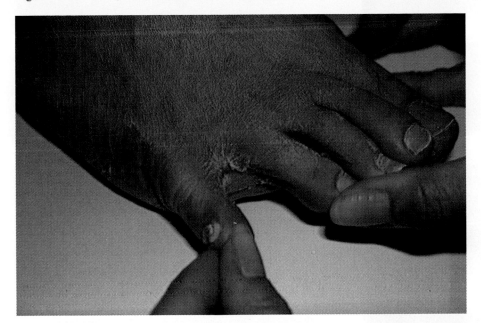

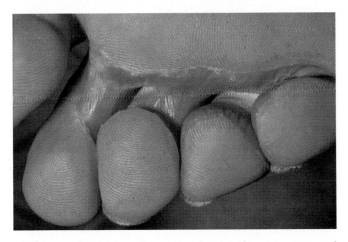

Figure 2.30 Interdigital tinea pedis. Exudative, macerated lesions.

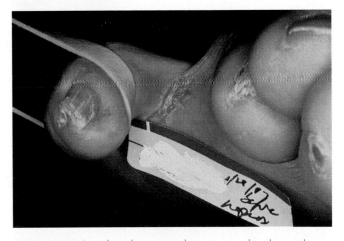

Figure 2.31 Interdigital tinea pedis associated with onychomycosis.

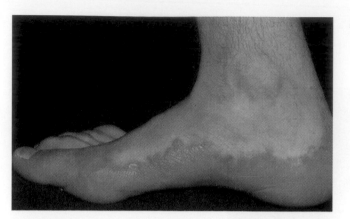

Figure 2.32 Moccasin-type tinea pedis.

Figure 2.33 Plantar and hand involvement in the same patient.

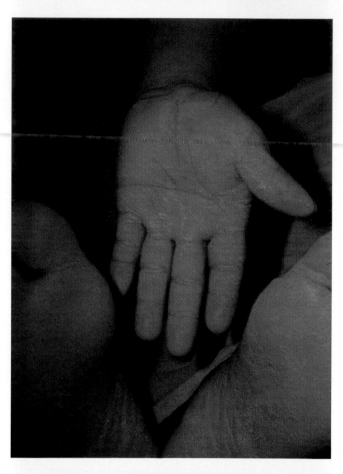

Figure 2.34 Moccasin-type tinea pedis usually associated with toenail infection.

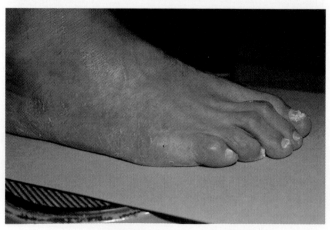

Figure 2.35 Vesiculobullous-type tinea pedis.

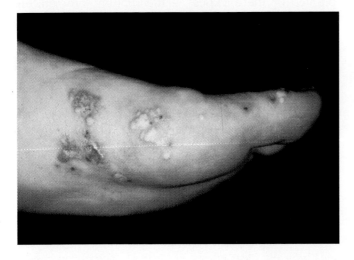

Figure 2.36 Vesiculopustular-type tinea pedis.

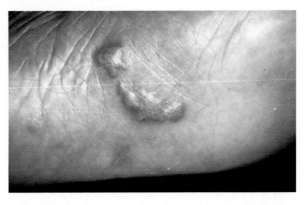

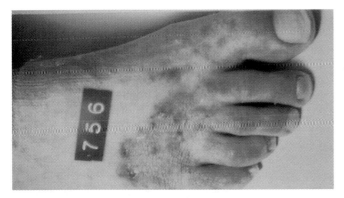

Figure 2.37 Vesiculobullous-type tinea pedis.

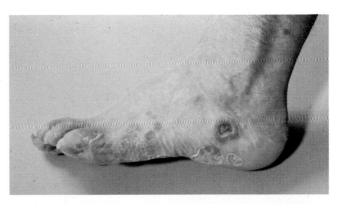

Figure 2.38 Ulcerative type of tinea pedis. *Trichophyton rubrum*, *Candida albicans*, and *Staphylococcus aureus* were isolated.

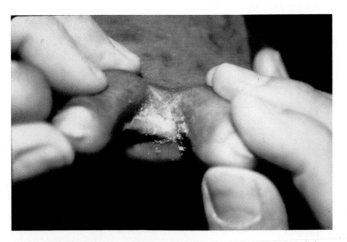

Figure 2.39 Tinea pedis. Interdigital type due to *Scytalidium dimidiatum*. The lesions are indistinguishable from those caused by dermatophytes. (Courtesy of Dr. Donald Greer.)

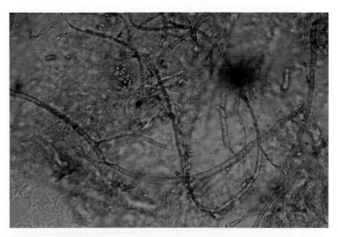

Figure 2.40 A KOH preparation from tinea pedis infected with *Scytalidium dimidiatum*. Note the dark pigmented hyphae. (Courtesy of Dr. Donald Greer.)

tive, culture is warranted. The standard medium for culturing dermatophytes is Sabouraud's dextrose agar containing cycloheximide and an antibacterial antibiotic.

Treatment   Two parameters should be considered in determining cure of a fungal infection (Table 2.4): (1) clinical cure with reduction in erythema, scaling, and so forth and (2) mycologic cure evaluated by KOH preparations and cultures. Total cure can be achieved only when both criteria are met.

Interdigital Toe Web Infections   Typical agents such as allylamines, imidazoles, and ciclopirox olamine are beneficial.[19] The imidazoles and ciclopirox olamine have an additional advantage because of their anticandidal and antibacterial activity.[20] Since bacteria are often involved in the macerated and erosive type of tinea pedis, broad-spectrum topical antifungal agents should be the first line of therapy. Tolnafate has little effect on *Candida* and bacteria.[20]

Table 2.4 Prescription and Over-the-Counter Topical Antifungal Products

GENERIC NAME	DRUG CLASS
Prescription products	
Griseofulvin	
Ciclopirox	
Haloprogin	
Clotrimazole	Imidazole derivatives
Miconazole	
Econazole	
Ketoconazole	
Oxiconazole	
Sulconazole	
Itraconazole	Triazoles
Fluconazole	
Naftifine	Allylamines
Terbinafine	
Butenafine	
Over-the-counter products	
Tolnaftate	
Miconazole	
Clotrimazole	
Undecylenic acid	
Gentian violet	
Whitfield's ointment	

Plantar, Moccasin-Type Tinea Pedis   Treatment is complicated by the thickness of the stratum corneum, the relatively low immunogenicity of *T. rubrum,* and involvement of the nails. Combined systemic and topical therapy followed by long-term use of topical therapy can contain the process. Itraconazole and oral terbinafine seem promising.[21,22]

Vesiculobullous Tinea Pedis   Acute vesicular lesions should be treated as any acute dermatitis. Compresses with Burow's solution and topical corticosteroids coupled with systemic antifungal therapy are sufficient for acute attacks. The fungicidal allylamines appear to be the best choice.

Prognosis   Uncomplicated tinea pedis usually responds to topical and systemic therapy. Bullae and vesicles typically clear after a short time. The chronic moccasin type is the most difficult to eradicate. This type is usually associated with onychomycosis. Systemic treatment combined with topical antifungal agents is recommended to treat both nail infection and tinea pedis to avoid relapses.

Differential Diagnosis   The differential diagnosis of tinea pedis includes toe cleft impetigo induced by bacteria or *Candida,* contact dermatitis, pustular psoriasis (Figs. 2.41 and 2.42) interdigital intertrigo (Fig. 2.43) idiopathic hyperkeratosis, erysipelas, pitted keratolysis, and fixed drug reaction. Erythrasma of the toe web is particularly difficult to differentiate from intertriginous tinea pedis. Wood's light shows the coral red fluorescence characteristic of erythrasma, ruling out tinea pedis.

Onychomycosis

Onychomycosis is an infection of the nail by fungi. Any part of the nail unit may be invaded by fungi: hyponychium, nail bed, nail matrix, nail plate, and nail folds. The etiologic agents may be determined by KOH preparation and a fungal culture. After ascertaining the diagnosis, the physician can choose from a wide variety of therapeutic options. Several factors to consider before selecting a therapy are patient compliance, dosage schedule, potential drug interactions, causative agents, extent of onychomycotic involvement, and cost of treatment. Oral griseofulvin and ketoconazole are old, well-recognized therapeutic agents; itraconazole, terbinafine, and fluconazole are new oral agents now available for the treatment of onychomycosis. These novel agents seems to be safe, and they will overtake griseofulvin as the drug of choice in the oral treatment of nail infections. Alternatives to systemic management of onychomycosis include topical and

Figure 2.41 The vesiculopustular eruption could be either psoriasis dyshidrosis or tinea. KOH was negative. Diagnosis is therefore psoriasis.

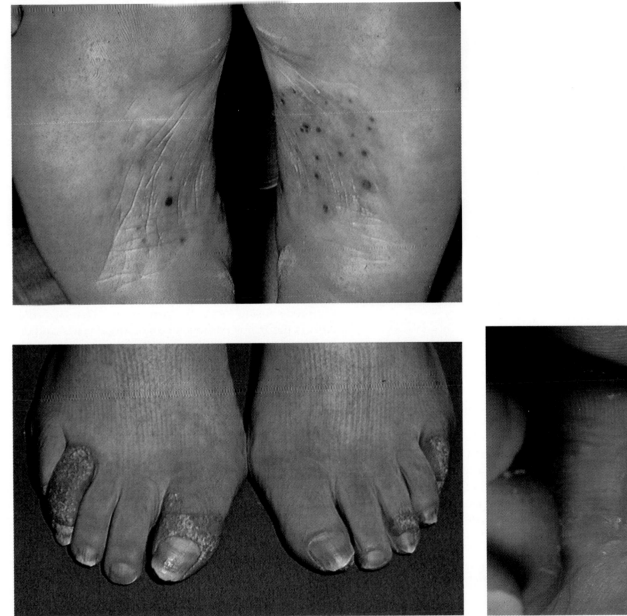

Figure 2.42 Hyperkeratosis of the toenails due to psoriasis.

Figure 2.43 Nonmicrobiologic toe web intertrigo. KOH was negative.

surgical treatments. The application of antifungal nail lacquer, for instance, may be effective topical therapy for the treatment of less severe forms of onychomycosis.

Etiology   Onychomycosis means fungal infection of the nail. This term includes infection due to dermatophytes, yeast, and nondermatophytic fungi. The common etiologic agents of onychomycosis are listed on the following page. Infection associated with dermatophytes are specifically defined as tinea unguium. Onychomyco-

sis occurs in approximately 2.7% of the general population, but it increases to almost 20% of the U.S. population between 40 and 60 years of age.[23] Mycotic infections of the nail resulting from dermatophytes account for more than 90% of the infections. Infections of the toenails is more common than infection of the fingernails, reflecting their association with higher prevalent tinea pedis. The wearing of shoes explains in part the overall higher incidence of fungal disease in the lower extremities. Onychomycosis occurs in all parts of the world.

MAJOR MICROORGANISMS OF ONYCHOMYCOSIS

Dermatophytes
- *Trichophyton rubrum*
- *Trichophyton mentagrophytes*
- *Epidermophyton flocussum*

Nondermatophytic Molds[a]
- *Aspergillus species*
- *Scopulariopsis brevicaulis*
- *Fusarium species*
- *Acremonium species*
- *Scytalidium dimidiatum[b]*
- *Scytalidium hyalinum[b]*

Yeast
- *Candida albicans*

[a] *It is important to perform a culture to distinguish molds from dermatophytes because molds may not respond to conventional therapy.*

[b] *Prevalent in tropical and subtropical regions.*

Clinical Features Onychomycosis is clinically classified into four types (Fig. 2.44, Table 2.5). Distal subungal onychomycosis is the most common type of nail infection; it is characterized by infection of the nail bed. Infection starts in the hyponychium with proximal spread. Nail involvement comes much later. Subungal hyperkeratosis causes lifting of the nail plate and onycholysis, resulting in crumbling and breakage of the nail (Fig. 2.45 and 2.46). Lateral onychomycosis is clinically similar to distal subungual onychomycosis except that it starts on the lateral edge of the nail plate (Fig. 2.47). This type of onychomycosis presents therapeutic problems.[24] *T. rubrum* is the leading dermatophyte isolated on culture.

Table 2.5 Classification of Onychomycosis

ROUTE OF INVASION	MICROORGANISMS
Distal subungual onychomycosis	Dermatophytes Nondermatophytic molds[a] Yeasts
Superficial white onychomycosis	Dermatophytes Nondermatophytic molds[a]
Proximal white subungual onychomycosis	Dermatophytes Yeasts
Candidal onychomycosis	Yeasts

[a] When nondermatophytes are suspected, media with and without cycloheximide should be included.

In white superficial onychomycosis, the fungus invades the nail plate directly, producing a crumbled white surface (Fig. 2.48). This clinical variety is unusual and is seen almost exclusively on toenails. *T. mentagrophytes* and species of *Aspergillus, Fusarium, Cephalosporium,* and *Acremonium* are typically recovered from these nails.

Proximal subungal onychomycosis is distinguished by fungal invasion under the cuticle leading to infection of the proximal nail bed and finally the nail plate (Fig. 2.49A). The nail plate remains intact and develops a white color near the cuticle. *T. rubrum* is the most common etiologic agent. Proximal white subungal onychomycosis is the rarest form of nail infection in the general population. This form has been associated with acquired immunodeficiency syndrome (AIDS) and is considered an early clinical marker of human immunodeficiency virus (HIV) infection.[25] The combination of proximal and distal involvement may lead to extensive nail dystrophy or a yellow-white opacity of the whole nail (Fig. 2.49B). Candidal onycholysis occurs where there is separation of the nail plate from the bed (Fig. 2.50). Occupational hand immersion in liquid is often the predisposing factor for paronychia. *Candida albicans* is the major pathogenic microorganism. Candidal onychomycosis (candidal granuloma) occurs mainly in patients with chronic mucocutaneous candidiasis and immunodeficient patients with invasion of the nail plate (Fig. 2.51).

Diagnosis In patients with distal subungal onychomycosis, the abnormal nail is clipped as proximally as possible with a nail clipper, and scrapings are taken from the nail bed (Fig. 2.52). Subungal keratinic debris can be obtained by using a small curet (Fig. 2.53). Nail plate clippings are not recommended for culture and KOH preparation; however, in the absence of subungal debris, nail plate clippings can be used if pulverized prior to direct microscopy and culturing (see Fig. 1.4). For proximal subungal onychomycosis, by using a scalpel blade, the normal surface of the nail plate in the lunular area is pared down to get to the ventral portion of the plate. The white material from deeper portions of the plate is collected. For white superficial onychomycosis, the white spots are scraped with a scalpel blade, discarding the outermost layers to avoid contamination. When both culture and KOH are negative, a nail biopsy is a last resort.

Two new diagnostic techniques, immunohistochemistry and flow cytometry, are useful in identifying different dermatophytes, yeasts, and nondermatophytic molds. Immunohistochemistry utilizes antibodies to discern certain fixed fungi from the background, and flow cytometry differentiates fungal cells on the basis of their molecular differences. These techniques provided further evidence that mixed infections do occur.[26]

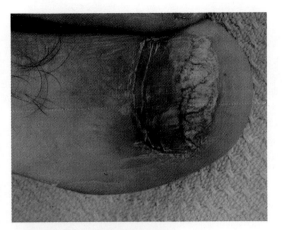

Figure 2.45 Distal subungual onychomycosis. Note thickening of the nail bed. *Trichophyton rubrum* was isolated.

Figure 2.44 Four patterns of nail infections demonstrating different entry points. (Courtesy of Janssen Pharmaceuticals.)

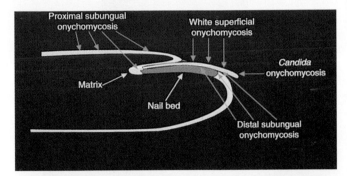

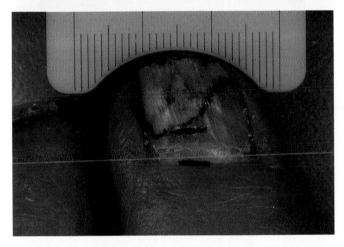

Figure 2.46 Distal subungual onychomycosis. *Trichophyton mentagrophytes* was isolated.

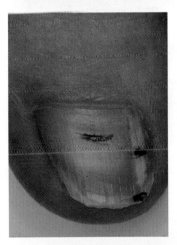

Figure 2.47 Lateral subungual onychomycosis. Infection starts at the lateral edge of the nail plate. *Trichophyton rubrum* was isolated.

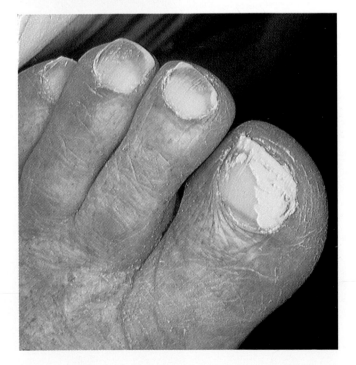

Figure 2.48 White superficial onychomycosis. The fungus invades the nail plate directly.

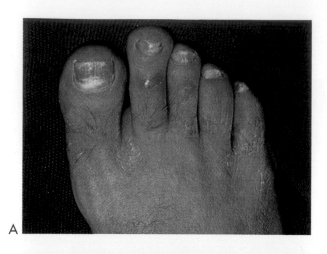

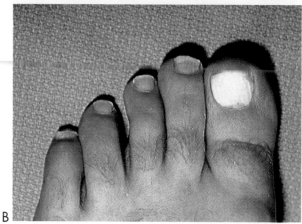

Figure 2.49 (A) Proximal subungual onychomycosis. *Trichophyton rubrum* is the most common etiologic agent. **(B)** Proximal and distal subungual onychomycosis in an AIDS patient. (Courtesy of Dr. Timothy Berger.)

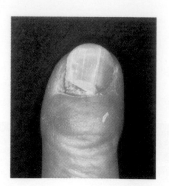

Figure 2.50 Candidal paronychia and onychomycosis. Note the proximal and paronychial involvement. (Courtesy of Dr. Richard Odon.)

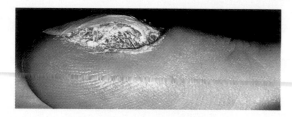

Figure 2.51 Candidal onychomycosis (granuloma) in a patient with mucocutaneous candidiasis.

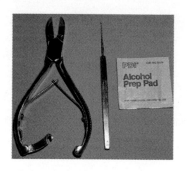

Figure 2.52 Nail clippers used to cut back the nail as proximal to the cuticle as possible. By treating the nail area with an alcohol pad, bacterial contamination is reduced.

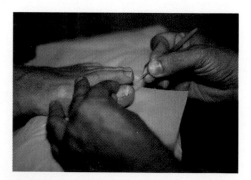

Figure 2.53 Nail debris is collected with a curet.

Table 2.6 Treatment Guidelines[a]

AGENT	ROUTE	DOSAGE	DURATION	SITE	SPECTRUM
Griseofulvin ultramicrosize	Oral	750 mg/day	12–18 mo	Toenail	Narrow[b]
		750 mg/day	6–9 mo	Fingernail	
Ketoconazole[c]	Oral	200–400 mg/day	8–18 mo	Toenail	Broad[d]
		200–400 mg/day	4–6 mo	Fingernail	
Itraconazole	Oral	200 mg/day	3–4 mo	Toenail	Broad
		400 mg/day (pulse)[e]	7 days; 1 wk/mo for 3–4 mo		
		200 mg/day or 400 mg/day (pulse)	6 wk for 2 mo	Fingernail	
Fluconazole[e]	Oral	150 mg/wk (pulse)	9–12 mo	Toenail	Broad
			3–6 mo	Fingernail	
Terbinatine	Oral	250 mg/day	3–4 mo	Toenail	Broad
		250 mg/day	6 wk	Fingernail	

[a] Many relapses of onychomycosis are caused by recurrence of tinea pedis and reinfection of the nail bed. Therefore long-term management with topical antifungal agents to treat tinea pedis is recommended.

[b] Active against dermatophytes only.

[c] Because of hepatotoxicity, prolonged regimens are not recommended.

[d] Active against dermatophytes, yeasts, and some molds.

[e] Labeled indications in the United States do not include onychomycosis. Before using the drug, please consult an up-to-date reference for current indications, side effects, drug interactions, and dosage schedule.

Direct microscopy using 15 to 20% KOH should reveal either presence or absence of fungal elements. The preparation should be heated gently (without boiling) to dissolve keratinic materials. Dimethyl sulfoxide, when added to KOH, may enhance the procedure.

For cultures, Sabouraud's dextrose agar is the most frequently used medium to isolate dermatophytes.[27] The medium is available with and without selective antibiotics. When samples are taken from nail infections, both types are recommended to permit the isolation of nondermatophytic fungi. A 2- to 3-week period is required to grow fungi at room temperature.

Treatment

Systemic Therapy   Consult Table 2.6 for recommended treatment guidelines.

Griseofulvin, introduced in the late 1950s, was the first effective oral agent in dermatophytic infection. Its efficacy in fingernail infections was good, but its activity was disappointing in toenail infections.[28] Long-term therapy is required: 6 to 9 months' duration for fingernail infection and 12 to 18 months for toenail infections.

Ketoconazole became available in 1980. Because of its spectrum against dermatophytes, yeast and several

mold,[29] ketoconazole was initially considered as the ideal agent for onychomycosis, but the potential risk of hepatotoxicity has restricted its use. Because of this hazard, long-term monitoring is recommended when prescribing ketoconazole.

Itraconazole is a broad-spectrum synthetic antifungal. It is highly lipophilic and virtually insoluble in water. The drug is delivered to the nail plate via the nail matrix and the nail bed. Therapeutic drug concentrations persist within affected fingernails for 6 months and within toenails for 9 months after the drug therapy is stopped.[30] Based on the nail pharmacokinetics, two dosage regimens are recommended for the treatment of nail disease. The first is a continuous regimen of 200 mg for 3 months in toenail infection and for 6 weeks in fingernail disease.[31] Pulse dosing of 1 week on and 3 weeks off for 3 to 4 months has shown efficacy equal to continuous therapy.[30,32] Intermittent therapy should reduce the cost of treatment and may increase patient compliance. Itraconazole should be given with food. Because of its broad activity, itraconazole may be effective in the treatment of onychomycosis due to nondermatophytes.

Fluconazole is a water-soluble, broad-spectrum antifungal agent. Because of its pharmacokinetics, flucona-

Figure 2.54 Infection of the nail due to *Scytalidium dimidiatum*. *Scytalidium* causes infection in both the nail and foot. (Courtesy of Dr. Donald Greer.)

Figure 2.55 Infection of the nail due to *Scopulariopsis brevicaulis*. (Courtesy of Dr. Donald Greer.)

Figure 2.56 Toenail in a patient with psoriasis. Note pits in the nail plate.

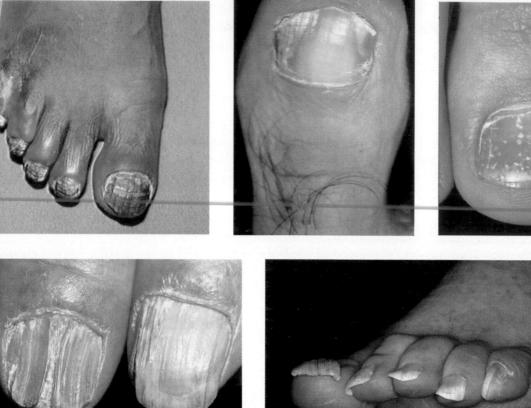

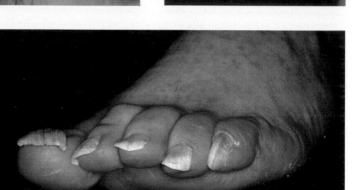

Figure 2.57 Nail changes in a patient with lichen planus. Increased longitudinal striations are common.

Figure 2.58 Onychogryphosis. Note the abnormal curvature of the nail plate. (Courtesy of Dr. Richard Odom.)

zole must be continued until the nail has completely grown out. The drug has been used in a dose of 150 mg once weekly for up to 9 months.[33] Fluconazole can be administered with or without food. Various doses are being investigated in the United States. Fluconazole is not currently approved by the Food and Drug Administration for the treatment of onychomycosis in the United States.

Terbinafine is fungicidal and highly lipophilic and concentrates in the stratum corneum, in sebum, and in hair follicles. The drug is active against dermatophytes and some species of *Candida*. Terbinafine persists in the nail plate up to 4 months after therapy is discontinued. Tinea unguium responds remarkably well to terbinafine given orally in doses of 250 mg/day for 12 to 16 weeks.[34] Intermittent therapy with 500 mg of terbinafine daily for 1 week every month for 4 months was quite effective in toenail infection.[35]

Topical Therapy   Most topical antifungal agents have little value as primary therapy in the majority of cases of onychomycosis. Many topical agents are useful in preventing the relapse of chronic tinea pedis, which often accompanies onychomycosis. This step hence may limit the possibility of reinfection of nails. The concomitant use of topical therapy with newer oral agents is promising.

For either topical or systemic treatment, nail avulsion has shown to reduce significantly the treatment period for onychomycosis. Nail avulsion may be performed either surgically or chemically. Urea ointment under occlusion will remove only the diseased portion of the nail, leaving the normal nail intact.

Prognosis   Fingernail infection has a much better prognosis than toenail infection. After infection has cleared, the prophylactic treatment of the foot is required to discourage reinfection of the skin or nails. A 1-week pulse therapy with itraconazole just at the beginning of reinfection may be useful.

Differential Diagnosis   Infections due to nondermatophytic fungi, psoriasis, lichen planus, trauma, and onychogryphosis may mimic tinea unguium (Figs. 2.54 to 2.58). Dermatophytic infection must be definitively established to protect the patient from being mistakenly given long and expensive oral antifungal therapy.

REFERENCES

1. Palmer SR, Bass JW: Tinea nigra palmarius and plantaris: a black fungus producing black spots on the palms and soles. Pediatr Infect Dis 8:48, 1989

2. Carr JF, Lewis CN: Tinea nigra palmaris: treatment with thiabendazole topically. Arch Dermatol 111:904, 1975

3. Gip L: Black piedra: the first case treated with terbinafine. Br J Dermatol, suppl., 130:26, 1994

4. Kalter DC: Genital white piedra: epidemiology, microbiology and therapy. J Am Acad Dermatol 14:982, 1986

5. Wilmington M, Aly R, Frieden H: *Trichophyton tonsurans* tinea capitis in the San Francisco Bay area: increased infection demonstrated in a 20-year survey of fungal infections from 1974 to 1994. J Med Vet Mycol 34:285, 1996

6. Rosenthal SA, Vanbreuseghem R: Viability of dermatophyte in epilated hairs. Arch Dermatol 85:143, 1962

7. Bable DE, Baughman SA: Evaluation of the adult carrier in juvenile tinea capitis caused by *Trichophyton tonsurans*. J Am Acad Dermatol 21:1209, 1989

8. Gan VN, Petruska M, Ginsberg CM: Epidemiology and treatment of tinea capitis: ketoconazole vs. griseofulvin. Pediatr Infect Dis J 6:46, 1987

9. Tanz RR, Hebert AA, Eskerly NB: Treating tinea capitis: should ketoconazole replace griseofulvin? J Pediatr 112:987, 1988

10. Martinez-Roig A, Torres-Rodrigues JM, Barlett-Coma A: Double-blind study of ketoconazole and griseofulvin in dermatophytoses. Pediatr Infect Dis J 7:37, 1988

11. Degreef H. Itraconazole in the treatment of tinea capitis. Cutis 58:90, 1996

12. Haroon TS, Hussain I, Aman S et al: A randomised double-blind comparative study of terbinafine for 1, 2 and 4 weeks in tinea capitis. Br J Dermatol 135:86, 1996

13. Aly R, Berger T: Common superficial infections in patients with AIDS. Clin Infect Dis, suppl. 2, 22:S128, 1996

14. Rippon JW: Cutaneous infections. Dermatophytosis and dermatomycosis in medical mycology. The Pathogenic Fungi and the Pathogenic Actinomycetes (ed 3). Saunders, Philadelphia, 1988:69

15. Taplin D: Superficial mycoses. J Invest Dermatol 67:77, 1976

16. Leyden JJ, Aly R Tinea: Pedis Seminars in Dermatol 12:280, 1993

17. Hay RJ, Moore MK: Clinical features of superficial fungal infections caused by *Hendersonula toruloidea* and *Scytalidium*. Br J Dermatol 110:677, 1984

18. Frankel DH, Rippon J: *Hendersonula toruloidea* infection in man. Mycopathologica 105:175, 1989

19. Gupta AK, Sander DN, Shear NH: Antifungal agents: an overview. Part II. J Am Acad Dermatol 30:911, 1994

20. Lehser JL, Jr, Smith JG, Jr: Antifungal agents in dermatology. J Am Acad Dermatol 17:383, 1987

21. Hay RJ, Clayton YM, Moore MK, Midgely G: Itraconazole in the treatment of chronic dermatophytosis. J Am Acad Dermatol 23:561, 1990

22. Savin RC: Oral terbinafine vs. griseofulvin in the treatment of moccasin type of tinea pedis. J Am Acad Dermatol 23:807, 1990

23. Zais N: Onychomycosis. p. 445. In Daniel CRM (ed): Dermatologic Clinics. Saunders, Philadelphia, 1985

24. Baran R, Aly R: Onychomycosis: diagnosis and current treatments. In Aly R, Maibach H, Beutner K (eds): Cutaneous, Viral, Bacterial and Fungal Infections. Marcel Dekker, New York, in press

25. Aly R, Berger T: Common superficial fungal infections in patients with AIDS. Clin Infect Dis, suppl. 2, 22:S128, 1996

26. Pierard GE, Arresse JE, De Doncker et al: Present and potential diagnostic techniques in onychomycosis. J Am Acad Dermatol 34:273, 1996

27. Aly R: Culture media for growing dermatophytes. Am J Acad Dermatol 31:S107, 1994

28. Davies RR, Everall JD, Hamilton E: Mycological and clinical evaluation of griseofulvin for chronic onychomycosis. Br J Dermatol 3:364, 1967

29. Holub PG, Hubbard ER: Ketoconazole in the treatment of onychomycosis. J Am Podiatr Med Assoc 77:338, 1987

30. Willemsen M, De Doncker P, Willems J et al: Post-treatment itraconazole level in the nail: new implication for treatment in onychomycosis. J Am Acad Dermatol 26:731, 1992

31. Piepponen T, Blomquist K, Brand H et al: Efficacy and safety of itraconazole in the long-term treatment of onychomycosis. J Antimicrob Chemother 29:195, 1992

32. Odom R, Aly R, Scher RK et al: A multi-center, placebo-controlled, double-blind study of intermittent therapy with itraconazole capsules for the treatment of onychomycosis of the fingernail. J Am Acad Dermatol 36:231, 1997

33. Nahass GT, Siso M: Onychomycosis: successful treatment with once-weekly fluconazole. Dermatology 186:59, 1993

34. Baudraz-Rosselet F, Rakosi J, Wili PB et al: Treatment of onychomycosis with terbinafine. Br J Dermatol suppl. 29, 126:40, 1992

35. Tosti A, Piraccinin BM, Stinchi C et al: Treatment of dermatophytic nail infections: an open randomized study comparing intermittent terbinafine therapy with continuous terbinafine treatment and intermittent intraconazole therapy. J Am Acad Dermatol 34:595, 1996

CHAPTER 3

Candidiasis: Cutaneous and Systemic Infections

David T. Roberts

SUMMARY

Etiology   Infection caused by yeasts of the genus *Candida*, including *C. albicans*, *C. glabrata*, *C. parapsilosis*, *C. tropicalis*, *C. guilliermondii*, *C. kefyr*, and *C. krusei* generally arising from the commensal reservoir, except for genital candidiasis (sexual transmission is known to occur) and oral candidiasis (infants may acquire infection intrapartum from vaginally infected mothers). In all varieties of cutaneous disease, there is always an underlying factor.

Clinical Features   Congenital candidiasis (discrete yellow vesicopustules often on an erythematous base that develop shortly after birth); oral candidiasis (discrete white shiny patches on the surface of the tongue, gums, buccal mucosa, and pharynx); denture stomatitis (slight soreness that develops into angular cheilitis); candidal leukoplakia (adherent white plaque on the tongue or buccal mucosa); candidal intertrigo (erythematous skin with vesicles and pustules at the edge of lesions, with small satellite lesions); distal candidal nail infection (onycholysis and subungual hyperkeratosis); chronic paronychia (swelling of the posterior nail fold with cuticular detachment from the nail plate); genital candidiasis (white plaques of yeast with well-demarcated edge and satellite lesions)

Differential Diagnosis   Oral cancer, lichen planus, psoriasis of the vulva, lichen sclerosis et atrophicus, vulvar intraepithelial neoplasia, Paget's disease

Diagnosis   Clinically by appearance, or with laboratory confirmation in cases of chronic disease to determine appropriate long-term therapy

Treatment   Antifungal drugs of the azole, polyene, and allylamine groups

Candidal infection is variously referred to as *candidosis* or *candidiasis*. There is no clear agreement as to which is the favored term and either may be preferred in different countries. The International Society for Human and Animal Mycology uses *candidosis*, which is compatible with the suffix used in other fungal infections. However, both terms are correct and refer to infection caused by yeasts of the genus *Candida*. *Candida albicans* is the most common species causing infection, but other members such as *Candida glabrata*, *Candida parapsilosis*, *Candida tropicalis*, *Candida guilliermondii*, *Candida kefyr*, and *Candida krusei* are increasingly important pathogens, especially in patients who are immunosuppressed. *Candida* yeasts are commensal organisms found in the gastrointestinal tract of healthy humans. They have a much higher pathogenic potential than many other commensal organisms, however, and regularly cause problems when there is superficial or systemic intercurrent disease, plus congenital, iatrogenic, or acquired immunosuppression or inoculation of the organism into an unfamiliar site. Candidiasis represents a relatively complex change in the host-parasite relationship, and there are many factors that contribute to virulence.

ETIOLOGY

Candida species are members of the normal human flora and as such are harmless colonizers of the mucous membranes and digestive tract. *C. albicans* is the species most commonly isolated, but the distribution of species is variable between the mouth and the gut. *Candida* yeasts are found in the mouth and gut in around 50% of the population and colonize the vagina in up to 20% of asymptomatic females. They are rarely isolated from healthy skin.

It is generally accepted that candidal infection arises from the commensal reservoir rather than from other infected individuals. The exceptions to this rule are genital candidiasis where sexual transmission is known to occur and oral candidiasis in infants who may acquire infection. An understanding of this disturbance of the host-parasite relationship requires consideration of host defence and virulence. Epidermal surfaces defend themselves against microbial invasion in a variety of ways. These include epidermal proliferation, T-cell immunity, phagocytosis, antifungal properties of secretions, secretory immunoglobulins, and the presence of other microbial flora. The first two of these, epidermal proliferation and T-lymphocyte immune responses, are thought to be most relevant in the prevention of candidal infection. It is now well recognized that patients with defective T cells and low CD4 counts as seen in human immunodeficiency virus (HIV) infection readily develop both cutaneous and mucosal candidiasis.

In some forms of congenital chronic mucocutaneous candidiasis, there is an enormous proliferation of epidermal cells with gross thickening of the stratum corneum. It is not entirely clear whether the yeasts stimulate such epidermal proliferation or whether proliferation allows for yeast overgrowth. However, it has been noted that epidermal proliferation does occur in experimentally induced infection in animals.

Keratinocytes are known to be capable of phagocytosing yeast cells, and therefore defects in the keratin layer may allow for entry of infection, as does an alteration in the indigenous microbial flora secondary to antibiotic therapy. Cutaneous candidiasis therefore tends to arise in patients who have defective T-cell immunity, local disease that reduces the efficiency of the epidermal barrier, or other factors that allow for alteration of the microbial flora such as antibiotic therapy and diabetes mellitus.

Such reduction in host defenses must be accompanied by an ability of *Candida* yeasts to take advantage of diminished defenses by producing virulence factors. The first and essential step in this process is adhesion of the yeast to the epithelial site, which depends on surface components of the fungal cells having an affinity for epithelial receptors. Both the protein and polysaccharide moieties of yeast surface glycoproteins are known to bind with various components of the host membrane glycoproteins. The ability of yeast to form hyphae, the so-called yeast-mycelial shift, has long been considered to be the primary pathogenic mechanism, and there is some evidence that hyphal forms adhere more readily to epithelial surfaces. However, it is now recognized that the yeast form is capable of invasion and should not be considered to be only a commensal.

The degree and depth of yeast penetration and subsequent amount of hyphae formation is clearly dependent on a complex interplay of both defense and virulence mechanisms that are not clearly understood. In normal individuals, host defenses are nearly always victorious in this struggle. However, even sometimes subtle changes in host defenses allow infection to become established.[1]

Skin infection may occur in a variety of circumstances. Cutaneous candidiasis may present within a few hours of birth because of intrauterine or intrapartum transfer of infection. Both oral candidiasis and diaper dermatitis complicated by candidal infection are relatively common in infancy. Vulvovaginal candidiasis, interdigital candidiasis, and candidal nail infection are often seen in young adults, whereas candidal intertrigo most often occurs in the elderly, as does denture stomatitis secondary to candidal infection. Chronic mucocutaneous candidiasis consisting of infection of the oral and genital areas together with acral infection of varying severity occurs secondary to a number of syndromes, which may be congenital or acquired. All of them produce a defect in T-cell immunity to varying degrees. Candidiasis secondary to iatrogenic immunosuppression is much more often systemic rather than cutaneous. In all varieties of cutaneous disease, there is always an underlying factor, which may be serious systemic disease, relatively trivial skin disease, concomitant therapy, or occupational factors that allow the yeasts a portal of entry.

CLINICAL FEATURES

Congenital Candidiasis

In congenital candidiasis, discrete yellow vesicopustules, often on an erythematous base, develop either at or a few hours after birth. They are most often seen on the face, chest, and trunk and may spread quite alarmingly to involve the whole surface area in 24 hours. The condition results from intrauterine or intrapartum transfer of infection to an immature skin, and evidence of maternal vaginal candidiasis can be found in more than half of all cases. *C. albicans* is the usual pathogen and can be isolated from skin scrapings of pustules. The pustules do not persist for very long and desquamate prior to spontaneous resolution. Occasionally, however, the disease can become systemic, often in neonates with other problems, and then represents a serious, potentially life-threatening complication. Such babies should therefore be carefully observed in the hospital until all skin signs clear.

Candidiasis of the Mouth and Tongue

Oral Candidiasis (Oral Thrush, Acute Pseudomembranous Candidiasis) Candidal infection of the mouth is most prevalent in infancy and old age and in the terminally sick. Otherwise it tends only to occur in patients with serious underlying disease. Clinically the disease presents with discrete white shiny patches on the surface of the tongue, gums, buccal mucosa, and pharynx (Fig. 3.1). These white plaques

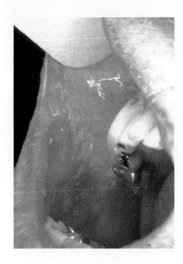

Figure 3.1 Oral candidiasis (thrush). (Courtesy of Dr. Timothy Berger.)

sometimes become confluent. They can readily be scraped off to reveal a raw erythematous base. White plaques that are easily removed in this way usually distinguish the lesions from other conditions, and the resulting specimen can be placed on a glass slide and sent to the laboratory, where yeast elements are readily visualized.

In a newborn infant, host defense mechanisms are immature, and infection may readily occur in nurseries through contact with toothbrushes, nurses' hands, and nipples. Infantile oral candidiasis may also be secondary to intrapartum infection in mothers with vaginal infection. There does not appear to be any relationship between oral candidiasis in infants and prematurity, low birth weight, and feeding methods.[2]

A similar picture is seen in patients following antibiotic therapy. Patients who receive antibiotics in combination for more serious forms of infection are probably more likely to develop oral thrush, while long-term antibiotic therapy for conditions such as acne rarely seems to give rise to oral candidiasis.

Denture Stomatitis (Denture Sore Mouth, Chronic Atrophic Candidiasis)

Although denture stomatitis is probably the most common disease associated with candidal infection, its recognition as such is relatively recent. However, the link between oral inflammation and the wearing of dentures is now firmly established.[3] Symptoms are relatively uncommon and may consist of only slight soreness, which is ignored by patients, who regularly present with angular cheilitis. In such cases, examination of the palate will often reveal erythema and edema of the hard palate that is in contact with the upper denture. Patients

who begin to wear dentures at a relatively young age regularly keep them in situ at all times. Elderly patients, on the other hand, who often have difficulty coming to terms with the discomfort of dentures, probably do remove them overnight more often but do not bother to leave them in a sterilizing solution and perhaps do not clean them assiduously either (Fig. 3.2). The inflammation would appear to be secondary to the occlusion of large numbers of yeasts in the space between the denture plate and the palatal epithelium. Defects in cell-mediated immunity in patients with denture stomatitis have not been identified.

Angular Cheilitis (Perleche)   Angular cheilitis is usually mentioned in descriptions of the various forms of oral candidiasis; however, it is by no means always or even regularly associated with candidal infection. It may be mechanical secondary to overclosure of the mouth in patients who either do not wear their dentures regularly or have old dentures that are worn down.

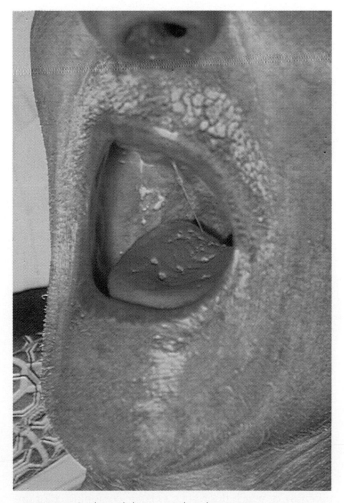

Figure 3.2 Oral candidiasis in edentulous patient.

Candidal Leukoplakia (Chronic Plaque-like Candidiasis, Chronic Hyperplastic Candidiasis)   Candidal leukoplakia consists of the appearance of a white plaque on the tongue or buccal mucosa that is notably adherent and cannot be scraped off as in acute oral candidiasis. It often appears in smokers, and histologically there is often atypia in the epithelial cells, and the condition may be preneoplastic. Occasionally a number of nodules develop within the plaque, and the condition is then sometimes known as chronic nodular candidiasis. Isolation of yeasts from these white plaques is probably not sufficient evidence to simply treat with antifungals, especially if the lesions do not resolve. A biopsy should certainly be arranged in any persistent or doubtful cases to exclude neoplastic change.

Midline Glossitis (Median Rhomboid Glossitis)   Midline glossitis is a chronic lozenge or rhomboid-shaped area on the dorsal surface of the tongue. This is a chronic condition and the role of *Candida* in its pathogenesis is unclear, although yeasts can readily be cultured in scrapings taken from the surface.

Other Forms of Oral Candidiasis

Any intraoral disease that interferes with epithelial barrier function may be superinfected by *Candida*. Thus culture of yeasts from abnormal mouths may not necessarily indicate a causal relationship. Examples of such diseases are oral lichen planus, papillary hyperplasia, fistulas, oral ulceration, and abscesses.

Candidiasis of the Skin and Nails

Candidal Intertrigo (Flexural Candidiasis)   The majority of cases of candidal intertrigo are secondary to *C. albicans,* which may cause disease in the groin area (Fig. 3.3), submammary (Fig. 3.4) and lower abdominal skin folds, axilla, and interdigital spaces.[4] The area is generally erythematous, and both vesicles and pustules are noted often toward the edge of lesions. Small satellite lesions outside the confluent area of infection are often diagnostic features. Typical patients are often obese, middle-aged, and diabetic.

Candidal infection of the toe clefts may be confused with and indeed is most often secondary to dermatophyte infection. Primary candidiasis of the toe webs is often noted in paraplegics who have neither sensation nor movement in their feet (Fig. 3.5). An important differential diagnosis in this site as well as in the groin and axilla is erythrasma, which fluoresces a classic coral pink color under Wood's light. Candidiasis of the finger webs, or erosio interdigitis blastomycetica, produces a typical white fissure in the finger webs with surrounding erythema (Fig. 3.6). It is not common and is usually of occupational origin. It appears in hairdressers, bartenders, and cooks among others who have wet occupations and are also subject to interdigital trauma, which allows a portal of entry for yeasts.

Diaper Dermatitis   Diaper dermatitis is a primary irritant reaction seen in the diaper area of infants. It is generally accepted that urease enzymes in feces release ammonia from urine, and this chemical has an acute irritant effect. It is therefore seen most commonly and severely in infants whose wet and dirty diapers are not changed as regularly as they should. The acute inflammatory skin reaction reduces epidermal barrier function and allows an easy portal of entry for *Candida,* which is present in feces.[5] The classic clinical picture is of white plaques on an erythematous base together with satellite lesions.

Candidal Nail Infection   Yeasts play a causal role in only 5 to 10% of all cases of onychomycosis. Three clinical varieties of candidal nail infection are recognized: distal candidal nail infection, candidal paronychia, and chronic mucocutaneous candidiasis.[6] The causal role of yeasts in the first two of these is controversial, and only in chronic mucocutaneous candidiasis is the pathogenic role of *Candida* universally accepted.

Distal nail dystrophy presents with onycholysis and subungual hyperkeratosis and is very difficult to distinguish from a dermatophyte infection (Fig. 3.7) Such cases are usually diagnosed when nail clippings and subungual scrapings are submitted for mycologic examination to exclude a dermatophyte infection and yeasts are reported on both microscopy and culture. *C. albicans* is the most common pathogen, followed by *C. parapsilosis*. There are, however, subtle differences in both the clinical appearance and history that are inconsistent with the diagnosis of a dermatophyte infection. Although the nail is onycholytic and subungual hyperkeratosis is present, there is often not the same degree of nail destruction as is seen in dermatophyte infection, and this may be related to the less potent keratolytic activity of yeasts. Fingernails are nearly always involved, whereas 80% of dermatophyte infection affects the toenails. Finally, such patients often give a history of Raynaud's phenomenon. It may be that this relatively poor blood supply diminishes the host response sufficiently to allow yeast infection of the normal nail, but equally it may be that diminished blood flow results in onycholysis, thus creating a portal of entry for the microorganism. It is unclear which is the pathogenic mechanism and thus difficult to decide whether long-term systemic antiyeast therapy should be prescribed.

Figure 3.3 Perianal candidiasis.

Figure 3.4 Submammary intertrigo with secondary candidal infection.

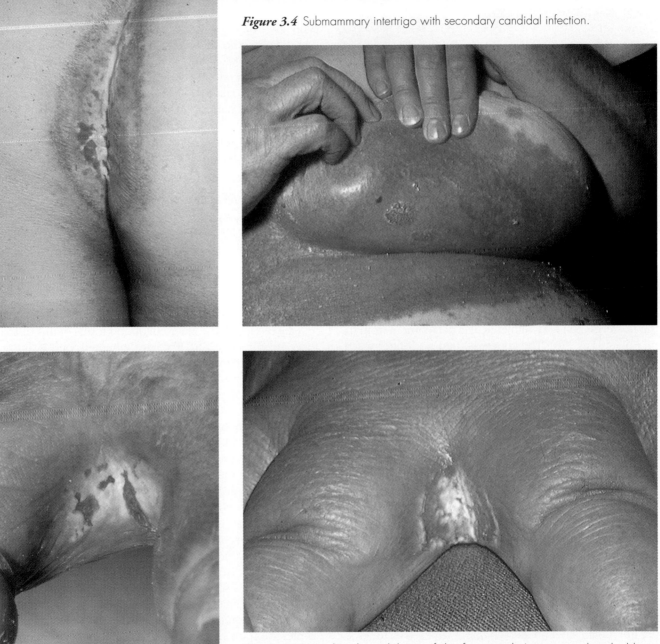

Figure 3.6 Interdigital candidiasis of the finger web (erosio interdigitalis blasto-mycetica).

Figure 3.5 Interdigital candidiasis in a para-plegic patient.

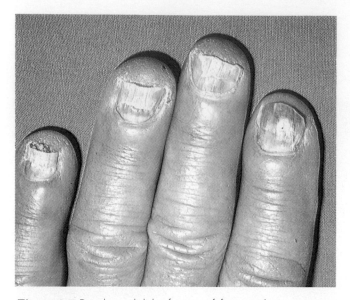

Figure 3.7 Distal candidal infection of fingernails in a patient with Raynaud's phenomenon.

Chronic paronychia initially presents as swelling of the posterior nail fold with cuticular detachment from the nail plate (Fig. 3.8). The cuticle is then no longer watertight and allows microorganisms to wash into the subcuticular space (Fig. 3.9). This in turn gives rise to further swelling of the posterior nail fold and further cuticular detachment. This vicious circle leads to increasing infection and ultimately a proximal nail dystrophy secondary to infection of the area in the nail matrix (Fig. 3.10). Both yeasts and bacteria infect the subcuticular space, and both may also be causal in the nail dystrophy.[7] The pathogenic role of *Candida* is therefore unclear. Some authorities believe that the primary event is related to a contact allergy to foodstuffs, producing an acute dermatitis reaction in the posterior nail fold, whereas others feel that any wet occupation will produce such changes in an irritant fashion (Fig. 3.11). Again the choice of treatment, which may be anti-inflammatory, anti-infective, topical, or systemic, remains controversial.

Chronic mucocutaneous candidiasis (described in greater detail later in the chapter) gives rise to gross thickening and hyperkeratosis of involved nails, which are heavily contaminated with *Candida* yeasts, again mainly *C. albicans*. The clinical picture is typical in full-blown cases and is accompanied by the other common manifestations of this disease.

Genital Candidiasis

Candidal vulvitis is invariably associated with candidal vaginitis. Patients present with an erythematous vulva on which are scattered typical white plaques of yeast (Fig. 3.12). The lesions often have a relatively well demarcated edge with the typical satellite lesions (Fig. 3.13). Pustules and vesicles are seen around the edge of the lesion in most acute cases.[8] Severe clinical candidal vulvitis is only an occasional accompaniment of vaginal candidiasis, and it is likely that other factors such as diabetes or local irritants such as occlusive underwear play a part in pathogenesis.

Candidal balanitis is nearly always seen in males whose sexual partner has vaginal candidiasis[9] (Fig. 3.14), and neither candidal vulvitis nor candidal balanitis should be diagnosed and treated in isolation without excluding vaginal candidiasis in either patient or sexual partner.

Chronic Mucocutaneous Candidiasis

Chronic mucocutaneous candidiasis is a rare syndrome that usually presents in early life with recurrent oral cutaneous and nail infections that usually prove notably recalcitrant and recurrent (Fig. 3.15). Candidiasis is often accompanied by other chronic viral and fungal skin infections (Fig. 3.16). Four childhood forms of this disease have been recognized. Two are inherited; one is autosomal recessive, and the other is autosomal dominant. The third form is associated with a polyendocrinopathy syndrome, and patients usually have hypoparathyroidism, hypoadrenalism, and sometimes hypothyroidism. Finally, an idiopathic variety occurs in children where none of the above apply. Adult forms usually occur in association with thymoma or systemic lupus erythematosus.[10] Associated defects in cell-mediated immunity are variable in both individual patients and with time. The disease may run a relatively benign course, with mild but chronic candidal infection, or may be severe, with associated systemic viral and pulmonary infections that often lead to early death. Investigations should certainly exclude endocrine disease, autoimmune disease, and thymomas, all of which may be treatable. Tests of immune function are nearly always carried out and may identify abnormalities, but of course these are generally irremediable, and treatment should be centered on prophylaxis of infection if this is possible.

Secondary Candidiasis

Although *Candida* yeasts are commensal organisms, they secondarily infect primary dermatologic diseases only rarely. However, patients with chronic psoriasis affecting the flexures (Fig. 3.17) and nails (Fig. 3.18) are prone to yeast overgrowth. Isolation of yeast from such sites should not be assumed to be causal, and treatment requires a combined approach aimed at both primary and secondary problems.

Figure 3.8 Chronic paronychia showing swelling of posterior nails folds.

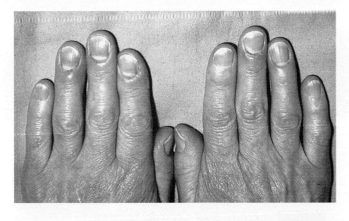

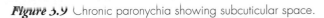

Figure 3.9 Chronic paronychia showing subcuticular space.

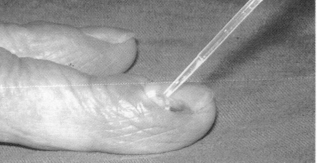

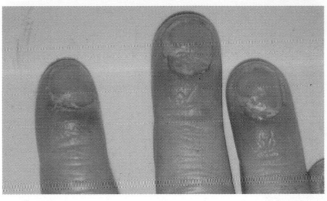

Figure 3.10 Chronic paronychia with proximal nail dystrophy.

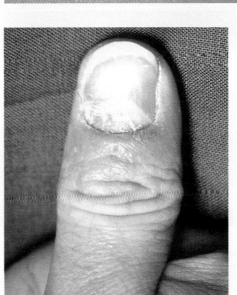

Figure 3.11 Chronic dermatitis of posterior nail fold with secondary candidal infection.

Figure 3.12 Candidal vulvitis.

Figure 3.13 Genital candidiasis spreading to the perianal area.

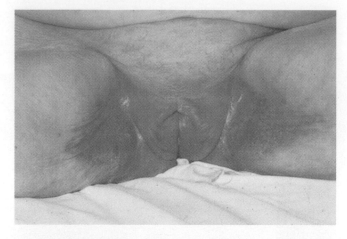

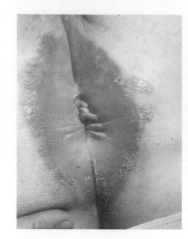

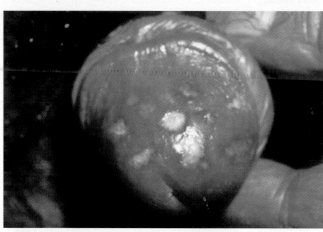

Figure 3.14 Candidal balanitis. (Courtesy of Dr. Timothy Berger.)

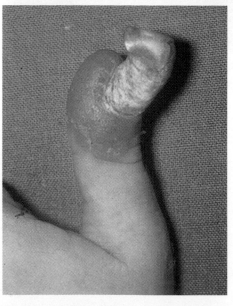

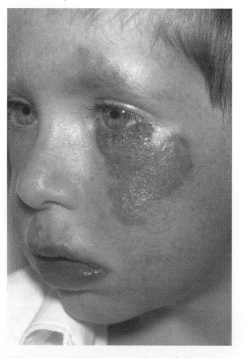

Figure 3.15 Candidal nail dystrophy in chronic mucocutaneous candidiasis.

Figure 3.16 Cutaneous candidiasis in chronic mucocutaneous candidiasis.

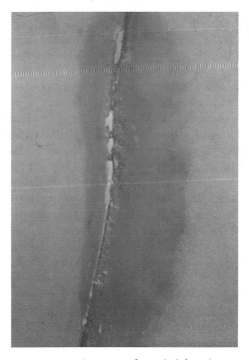

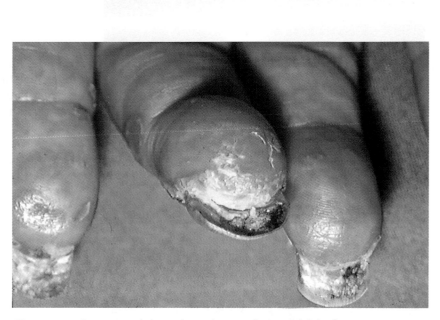

Figure 3.17 Psoriasis of natal cleft with secondary candidal infection.

Figure 3.18 Psoriatic nail dystrophy with secondary candidal infection.

Systemic Candidiasis

Systemic candidiasis almost always occurs in patients who have acquired or iatrogenic immunodeficiency and is becoming more prevalent with the increasing number of patients predisposed to infection.[11] The disease is more properly referred to as disseminated candidiasis, which more accurately describes the situation whereby yeasts spread to those sites where they are not normally commensal organisms. As in cutaneous candidiasis, *C. albicans* is the most frequently encountered species, although *C. tropicalis* is frequently seen in patients with granulocytopenia and *C. parapsilosis* is associated with parenteral nutrition. Almost any other *Candida* species may also cause disease in immunocompromised patients, even though they are hardly ever pathogenic in immunocompetent patients.

Pulmonary candidiasis occurs following hematogenous spread of yeasts and can only be diagnosed accurately antimortem by means of a lung biopsy and histopathologic examination. Chest x-ray appearances are nonspecific, and both serology and sputum culture are unreliable indicators. These patients are often very sick by the time infection is acquired, and speculative treatment may be required.

Candidal meningitis is uncommon and predominantly seen in newborn infants with systemic candidiasis. Candidal encephalitis is usually metastatic and nearly always diagnosed postmortem.

Candidal endophthalmitis (Fig. 3.19) may occur following hematogenous spread and appears to be more frequently encountered in heroin addicts. The diagnosis can sometimes be made by vitreous sampling.

Hepatic and hepatosplenic candidiasis may occur as part of generalized infection but may also be discovered in leukemic patients following remission-induction treatment (Figs. 3.20 and 3.21). Again, histology is required to confirm infection.

Candidal peritonitis may complicate peritoneal dialysis, gastrointestinal perforation, and abdominal surgery where yeasts can be cultured from ascitic fluid.

Candiduria may be transient and asymptomatic. Occasionally candidal cystitis and secondary renal candidiasis can occur following the hematogenous dissemination from the gastrointestinal tract, and yeast infection is suspected when there are elevated yeast counts in urine specimens obtained by suprapubic aspiration, positive blood cultures, and positive precipitant test. Sometimes yeast abscesses occur in the renal cortex, and so-called fungus balls, which are "compact masses of fungal filaments" develop in the renal pelvis.

Cardiac infection most frequently takes the form of an endocarditis. Preexisting valvular disease predisposes to this condition. The signs are similar to those of bacterial endocarditis.

Figure 3.22 Oral lichen planus.

Figure 3.23 Vulvar psoriasis.

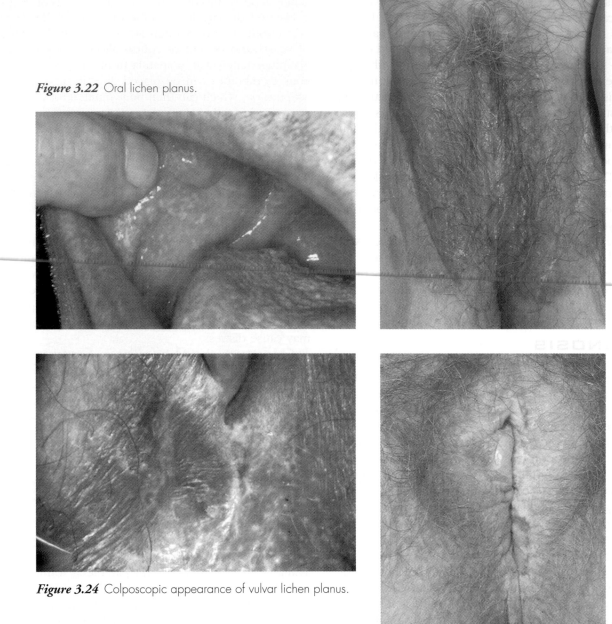

Figure 3.24 Colposcopic appearance of vulvar lichen planus.

Figure 3.25 Lichen sclerosis et atrophicus.

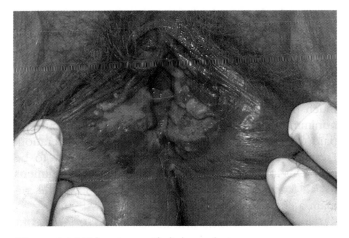

Figure 3.26 Vulvar intraepithelial neoplasia.

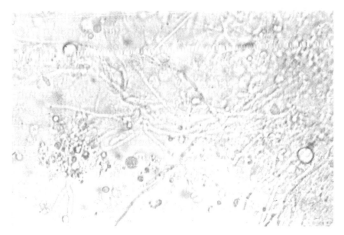

Figure 3.28 Potassium hydroxide direct microscopy of cutaneous candidiasis. (Courtesy of Dr. M.D. Richardson.)

azoles, polyenes, or allylamines are effective over relatively short treatment durations of up to 4 weeks. There are a number of proprietary combined preparations available: clotrimazole with hydrocortisone; miconazole with hydrocortisone; nystatin with hydrocortisone and clioquinol; clobetasone butyrate, nystatin, and oxytetracycline; and betamethasone diproprionate and clotrimazole. In addition, many physicians use their own mixtures, which, although not as stable as proprietary preparations, allow for potentially more accurate dilutions of the topical steroid.

Cutaneous candidiasis and infected diaper dermatitis in infants should be treated carefully in terms of the strength of topical steroid selected because of the danger of steroid absorption, and special attention should be paid to eradication of the underlying cause of the problem.

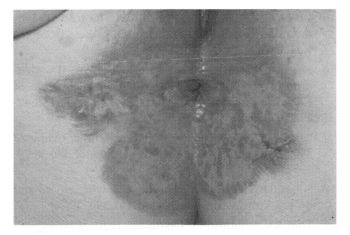

Figure 3.27 Perianal Paget's disease.

Oral Candidiasis

Uncomplicated oral candidiasis may be successfully treated topically with either nystatin (suspension or pastilles), amphotericin B (lozenges), or miconazole oral gel. In infants, the suspension or oral gel is preferable. Patients with denture stomatitis can be similarly treated, although it must be emphasized that they should both remove and place their dentures in a sterilizing solution overnight.

Candidal Nail Infection

Patients with distal nail dystrophy in whom *Candida* has been identified both on microscopy and culture with a high percentage of positive inocula should be treated systemically with itraconazole. Large studies to establish dosage regimen and treatment duration are lacking in the literature, but on theoretic grounds, itraconazole in a dosage of 200 mg daily for 6 weeks in fingernail infection or itraconazole in a dosage of 400 mg daily for 1 week per month repeated three times should be adequate.[16] Patients should however be warned that reversion of the nail to normal cannot be guaranteed, as it can never be certain that the candidal infection was the primary cause of the nail dystrophy. Chronic paronychia without proximal nail dystrophy probably does not require systemic antifungal treatment. A reasonable treatment regimen consists of a potent topical steroid together with an antiseptic such as betamethasone and clioquinol applied to the posterior nail fold together with the alternating once daily application of an imidazole lotion such as clotrimazole or miconazole applied to the proximal portion of the nail and an antibacterial

Treatment

There are numerous topical treatments.[4,5] However, depigmentation will remain for several months after treatment, and it is important to tell the patient. The patient should treat the whole trunk, neck, arms, and legs down to the knees even when small areas are involved. An inexpensive, effective, and cosmetically acceptable treatment is to use propylene glycol (50% in water),[6] which when applied twice daily for 2 weeks gives excellent results and little risk of skin irritation. Another treatment is to use ketoconazole as a cream[7] or in a foam solution.[8] Topical application of bifonazole, clotrimazole, econazole, or miconazole once or twice daily for 2 weeks is also effective.[4,5] Another effective treatment is zinc pyrithione shampoo[9] applied to affected areas after showering, left for approximately 5 minutes, and then rinsed off. This procedure should be repeated nightly for 2 weeks. Selenium sulfide is also effective, but the patient sometimes complains about the offensive odor and stinging sensation on the skin after application.[4,5]

Ciclopirox olamine (0.1% solution) applied once daily for 4 weeks was effective in 86% of 90 treated patients at a follow-up visit 4 weeks after the last day of treatment.[4,5] Terbinafine, an orally and topically active allylamine antifungal derivative, is orally active primarily against dermatophytes. It has been effective in the treatment of pityriasis versicolor in a 1% cream formulation applied topically once daily for 4 weeks[4,5]; 100% were cleared in the terbinafine group after 4 weeks in a single, blind, comparative study against bifonazole 1% cream.

Systemic therapy is primarily indicated for extensive lesions, for lesions resistant to topical treatment, and for frequent relapse. However, with short-term treatment, the risk of side effects with systemic therapy may be minimized, and oral antifungals may therefore be used even for other indications. Ketoconazole is an effective oral drug, with a broad antimycotic spectrum.[4,5,10] Overall, results have shown cure rates of 92% with a mean treatment period of 4 weeks.[10,11] However, with longer treatment periods, the risk for serious liver reactions, seen with oral ketoconazole, will increase.[10] Hay et al. have treated patients successfully with 200-mg tablets once daily for 5 days.[4,5] Rausch and Jacobs have shown that even one single dose of 400 mg may be effective.[4,5] The risk of side effects is minimized with short-term treatment.

Itraconazole, a triazole derivative, has been shown to be effective orally in well-conducted, controlled trials.[12] An effective treatment schedule is 200 mg daily for 5 to 7 days. The risk for serious side effects, especially liver toxicity, is much lower for itraconazole than for ketoconazole.

Fluconazole, a triazole derivative, has also been used in the treatment of pityriasis versicolor in a single dose of 400 mg.[4] Lesions in 17 of 23 patients (74%) were cleared 3 weeks after treatment, indicating that it is an effective alternative to other treatments. However, skin pharmacokinetic studies indicate that two doses given 1 week apart may be even more effective, and the patient compliance should still be high. The risk of side effects is low.

The high rate of recurrence, reaching 60% in 1 year and 80% after 2 years, is an outstanding problem. Recurrence is due to the presence of predisposing factors, which may be difficult to eradicate. A permanent cure is therefore difficult to achieve, which explains the chronicity. Consequently, a prophylactic treatment regimen is necessary to avoid recurrence. An effective prophylactic treatment is 200 mg of ketoconazole on 3 consecutive days every month.[11] Rausch and Jacobs have used a single dose of 400 mg ketoconazole every month as an effective prophylaxis in pityriasis versicolor.[4,5] Topically prophylactic treatment schedules may also be used, but the patient compliance is much lower.

Differential Diagnosis

Difficulties with differential diagnosis are due to the color of the lesions and the location. Diseases to consider include vitiligo (Fig. 4.8) and the pityriasis alba variant of atopic dermatitis. For pityriasis versicolor located in the groin and axilla, erythrasma and dermatophytosis are important. Psoriasis, seborrheic dermatitis, and confluent and reticulate papillomatosis are other dermatoses one should consider as differential diagnoses because they can coexist with pityriasis versicolor.

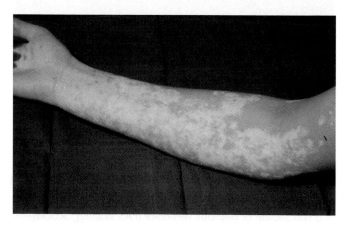

Figure 4.8 Vitiligo on the arm.

PITYROSPORUM (MALASSEZIA) FOLLICULITIS

Etiology

Pityrosporum (Malassezia) folliculitis is characterized by follicular papules and pustules localized to the back, chest, upper arm, sometimes the neck, and less often the face. It is often associated with a troublesome itching. The first well-documented study of *Pityrosporum* folliculitis was reported by Potter and co-workers in 1973.[4] This was later questioned, but several studies indicate that *P. ovale (M. furfur)* is the etiologic agent of *Pityrosporum* folliculitis.[4,13,14] Under the influence of predisposing factors, *Pityrosporum* folliculitis may be explained by an extensive growth following dominance of *P. ovale* in the hair follicle. Local occlusion may play an important role. The inflammation may be due both to products produced by the yeast and to free fatty acids produced as a result of the lipase activity of the fungus.

Clinical Features

The typical patient reports itching with follicular papules and pustules localized to the back, chest, upper arms, sometimes the neck, and more seldom the face (Figs. 4.9 and 4.10). The age of the patients with the disease varies between studies, but most of the patients are 30 years or older. We have in one study found a predominance of women with a ratio of 3:1, but in other smaller series this ratio was lower or reversed.[13] *Pityrosporum* folliculitis is

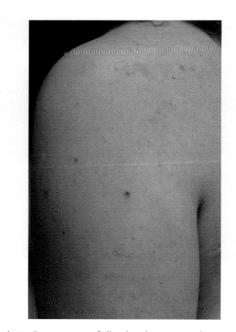

Figure 4.10 *Pityrosporum* folliculitis lesions on the upper arm.

more common in tropical countries, and one study from the Philippines has shown a prevalence of 16% in patients visiting a dermatologic clinic.[14] In temperate climates, the disease is more common during the summer months. Acne estivalis, with a clinical picture corresponding to *Pityrosporum* folliculitis, was originally described as a condition with heavy sun exposure. The disease is also seen as a complication in patients receiving oral corticosteroids or immunosuppressive treatment. It is also a complication seen more often in AIDS patients (see Ch. 7).

The typical lesions are small follicular papules and pustules. Pruritus is often the main complaint, and there is generally a discrepancy between the small lesions and the often troublesome itching. Distribution of lesions predominantly on the trunk, itching, and lack of comedones differentiate the condition from acne. However, the two diseases may often coexist, with nonitching acne lesions on the face and itching lesions of *Pityrosporum* folliculitis on the trunk and upper arms.

Pathology

If a biopsy is serial cut and methenamine silver stained, black, round, budding yeast cells and sometimes hyphae will be found in a dilated follicle (Fig. 4.11). Hyphae are only present in a minority of biopsies, but there are a tremendous number of blastospores.[13] There is an accumulation of mononuclear cells in and around the upper part of the follicle. In the superficial part of the

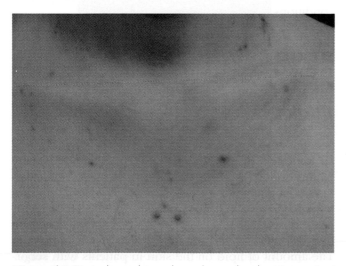

Figure 4.9 Typical papules and pustules on the chest in a patient with *Pityrosporum* folliculutis.

Pathology

The histologic picture is halfway between psoriasis and chronic eczema. In the epidermis, slight to moderate acanthosis and spongiosis can be found, and the horny layer shows focal areas of parakeratosis. A mild chronic inflammatory infiltrate is present in the dermis. The inflammatory cells are mainly T-helper cells[4,17,18] (Fig. 4.16).

Diagnosis

The diagnosis is based on the clinical criteria with typical lesions and distribution of the disease.

Treatment

Mild corticosteroid solutions, creams, or ointments are effective in the treatment of seborrheic dermatitis due to a nonspecific anti-inflammatory activity. However, they apparently have no effect on *P. ovale* because seborrheic dermatitis recurs quickly when corticosteroids are used, often within a few days after treatment has ended.

Antifungal therapy for *P. ovale* is effective in treating most cases of seborrheic dermatitis, and prophylactic treatment with antifungal drugs reduces the recurrence rate much more than corticosteroids[4,15,19] (Fig. 4.17). Ketoconazole is effective in vitro against *P. ovale,* with minimum inhibitory concentrations in the range of 0.02 to 0.5 μg/ml. Oral ketoconazole has been effective in a double-blind, placebo-controlled trial in patients with seborrheic dermatitis of the scalp and other areas.[4]

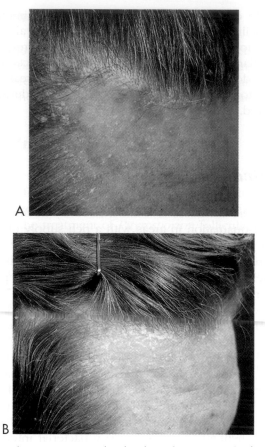

Figure 4.17 A patient with seborrheic dermatitis in the face and scalp before (A) and after (B) treatment with miconazole-hydrocortisone solution and cream. (Courtesy of Daktacort, Janssen Pharmaceutica.)

However, oral ketoconazole should be reserved for patients not responding to topical therapy. In another double-blind, placebo-controlled study, 2% ketoconazole cream has been effective in the treatment of seborrheic dermatitis of the scalp and face,[4] and in a comparative study between ketoconazole and hydrocortisone cream, no difference was seen in effectiveness.[4]

Ketoconazole shampoo used twice weekly is effective in treating seborrheic dermatitis of the scalp.[4] In a double-blind, placebo-controlled study of ketoconazole shampoo used twice weekly for 4 weeks, 89% of the ketoconazole group was cured, compared with only 14% in the placebo group. Ketoconazole used once weekly has also been effective in preventing recurrence of dandruff in previously treated patients.

Other topical antimycotics are effective in the treatment of seborrheic dermatitis[4,18,19]. Shampoos containing zinc pyrithione[4,15] or selenium sulfide[4,14] are effective. Propylene glycol solution has also been used successfully.

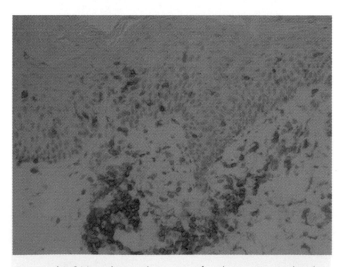

Figure 4.16 Histochemical staining of a skin section with seborrheic dermatitis showing an infiltrate in the dermis of predominantly T-helper cells.

Differential Diagnosis

Sometimes the differential diagnosis of atopic dermatitis and especially psoriasis localized in seborrheic areas may be difficult.

CONCLUSION

Today we have effective treatments for the more severe forms of these diseases. However, due to the presence of various predisposing factors, recurrence is a major problem in all three diseases, and a prophylactic treatment schedule is indicated to avoid this.

SUGGESTED READING

Albright S.D. Hitch J.M.: Rabbit treatment of tinea versicolor with selenium sulphide. Arch Dermatol 93:460, 1996

Faergemann J: Treatment of pityriasis versicolor with a single dose of fluconazole. Acta Derm Venereol 72:74, 1992

REFERENCES

1. Porro MN, Passi S, Caprill F, et al: Growth requirements and lipid metabolism of *Pityrosporum orbiculare.* J Invest Dermatol 66:178, 1976

2. Gordon MA: The lipophilic microflora of the skin. Mycologia 43:524, 1951

3. Faergemann J, Aly R, Maibach HI: Quantitative variations in distribution of *Pityrosporum orbiculare* on clinically normal skin. Acta Derm Venereol 63:346, 1983

4. Faergemann J: *Pityrosporum* infections. p. 69. In Elewski BE (ed): Cutaneous Fungal Infections. Igaku-Shoin, New York, 1992

5. Faergemann J: Tinea versicolor (pityriasis versicolor). p. 1. In Demis DJ (ed): Clinical Dermatology. Lippincott-Raven, Philadelphia, 1995

6. Faergemann J, Fredriksson T: Propylene glycol in the treatment of tinea versicolor. Acta Derm Venereol 60:92, 1980

7. Savin RC, Horwitz SN: Double-blind comparison of 2% ketoconazole cream and placebo in the treatment of tinea versicolor. J Am Acad Dermatol 15:500, 1988

8. Rekacewicz I, Guillaume JC, Benkhraba F, et al: A double-blind placebo-controlled study of a 2 percent foaming lotion of ketoconazole in a single application in the treatment of pityriasis versicolor. Ann Dermatol Venereol 117:709, 1990

9. Faergemann J, Fredriksson T: An open trial of the effect of a zinc pyrithione shampoo in tinea versicolor. Cutis 25:667, 1980

10. Jones HE: Ketoconazole today: a review of clinical experience. ADIS Press, Manchester, England, 1987

11. Faergemann J, Djärv L: Tinea versicolor: treatment and prophylaxis with ketoconazole. Cutis 30:542, 1982

12. Delescluse J: Itraconazole in tinea versicolor: a review. J Am Acad Dermatol 23:551, 1990

13. Back O, Faergemann J, Hörnqvist R: *Pityrosporum* folliculitis: a common disease of the young and middle-aged. J Am Acad Dermatol 12:56, 1985

14. Faergemann J, Johansson S, Back O: An immunologic and cultural study of *Pityrosporum* folliculitis. J Am Acad Dermatol 14:429, 1986

15. Shuster S: The aetiology of dandruff and the mode of action of therapeutic agents. Br J Dermatol 111:235, 1984

16. Faergemann J: Seborrhoeic dermatitis and *Pityrosporum orbiculare:* Treatment of seborrhoeic dermatitis of the scalp with miconazole-hydrocortisone (Daktacort), miconazole and hydrocortisone. Br J Dermatol 114:695, 1986

17. Bergbrant IM: Seborrhoeic dermatitis and *Pityrosporum ovale:* cultural, immunological and clinical studies. Acta Derm Venereol Suppl (Stockh) 167, 1991

18. Bergbrant IM, Johansson S, Robbins D, et al: An immunological study in patients with seborrhoeic dermatitis. Clin Exp Dermatol 16:331, 1991

19. Mathes BM, Douglass MC: Seborrheic dermatitis in patients with acquired immunodeficiency syndrome. J Am Acad Dermatol 13:947, 1985

CAUSATIVE ORGANISMS OF
MYCETOMA AND RELATIONSHIP TO
COLOR

Types of Grains

White

 Pseudallescheria boydii

 Acremonium species

 Nocardia organisms

Yellow to white

 Actinomyces israelii

 Nocardia caviae

Yellow to brown

 Streptomyces somaliensis

Black

 Madurella species

 Leptosphaeria senegalensis

Red

 Actinomadura pelletieri

Geographic Distribution   Both *Actinomyces* and *Nocardia* organisms are geographically widespread. *Nocardia* are soil organisms that produce disease when introduced into the skin through trauma. They may produce pulmonary disease when inhaled.

In a study in Mexico that covered over 2,100 cases in 30 years, males predominated (76%), and most of the patients were rural. Lower limbs were involved 64% of the time. *Actinomyces* caused 97.6%, with *N. brasiliensis* accounting for 86.6% and *A. madurae* 10%.[2] *Actinomadura pelletieri* is common only in Senegal and Chad. *S. somaliensis* causes 50% of the mycetomas in Somalia.

Clinical Features   The clinical features of mycetoma include those described above: swelling, draining sinuses, and grains. Most of these lesions are slowly developing and are painless. The swelling is rock hard and may resemble carcinoma because of the firmness and lack of early symptoms. The lesions are bound down to the bone, and indeed the bone may be involved.

Actinomycosis, also known as lumpy jaw, proceeds from necrotic oral tissue. This may accompany dental surgery, or may be the result of poor oral hygiene. The swelling is asymptomatic initially and develops into large swelling on the side of the jaw (Fig. 5.1). Eventually, draining sinuses appear and rupture, revealing the granules. The granules are sometimes known as grains or sclerotia. Often the granules are not visible initially and are only seen after a dressing is left in place. Examination of the dressing may be more helpful in this regard than examination of the patient.[3]

Although 65% of actinomycoses are cervical, smaller proportions are thoracic (from inhaled dental material) and abdominal-peritoneal (from swallowed material).

Primary cutaneous nocardial infections often arise from injuries in which soil-growing organisms are present (Fig. 5.2). There may be an initial verrucous papule, which may break down and ulcerate. Nodules along the course of draining lymphatics is one pattern

ease when necrotic material is present, such as following tooth extraction. Often the disease is produced concomitantly with other bacteria. The disease resembles a mycetoma because it consists of a swelling, draining sinuses, and grains.

The second is a group of aerobic soil organisms, including *Nocardia asteroides, Nocardia otitidis-caviarum,* and *Nocardia brasiliensis,* which produce skin disease by inoculation. These may become mycetoma or as ascending, sporotrichoid presentations. They can also cause pulmonary disease, usually characterized by draining sinuses. The organisms are characterized by their partial acid-fast staining.

The third group includes aerobic streptobacillary forms, including *Actinomadura madurae, Streptomyces somaliensis,* and others. They are also soil organisms and have produced actinomycotic mycetoma in varied locations.

Table 5.1 Characteristics of the Granules in Different Types of Mycetoma

	EDGE	CENTER	STAIN
Actinomycotic mycetoma	Branching 1–2 μm filaments; club-shaped ray at edge	Homogeneous	Gram-positive; Splendore-Hoeppli material at edge
Eumycotic mycetoma	Branching, septate hyphae, 4 μm or larger	Some have eosinophilic cement material	Gram positive
Botryomycotic mycetoma	Smooth eosinophilic material	Bacteria, cocci, or bacilli	Gram-positive or gram-negative; Splendore-Hoeppli material at edges and center

that may be produced. A tumor with draining sinuses is less often seen. Pulmonary nocardiosis probably originates as inhalation of airborne organisms. This may lead to pleural adhesions, fluid, and draining thoracic sinuses. The partially acid-fast nature of these organisms may lead to confusion when tuberculosis is suspected (Fig. 5.3). *Nocardia* species can also produce systemic disease, with involvement in more than one site, and central nervous system involvement. Dissemination is particularly evident in immunocompromised individuals[4] (Fig. 5.4).

The type of disease that develops and the progress may depend on the method of introduction. Experimental injection of BALB/c mice with *N. brasiliensis* in Freund's adjuvant produces disease rather quickly, while injection of the organisms alone produces disease after 6 months.[5]

Actinomycotic mycetoma produces classic mycetoma, often of extremities, with swelling, fibrosis, draining sinuses, and grains. This is a slowly developing, hard lesion with few symptoms. As with eumycotic mycetoma, the foot is most often involved (see below).

Pathology There is a dense fibrotic process with foci of granuloma. Within the granuloma, one notes purulent areas, and in the center of the polymorphonuclear leukocytes, the grains are visible. They are gram-positive and show radiating club-shaped filaments at the edge, surrounded by homogeneous eosinophilic material (Splendore-Hoeppli phenomenon).

Diagnosis The initial step in diagnosis is the isolation of the granule or grain. If the granule is colored, identi-

Figure 5.2 Primary cutaneous nocardiosis in the finger. (Courtesy of Dr. Nancy Warren.)

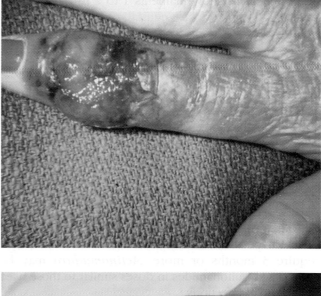

Figure 5.1 Actinomycosis or lumpy jaw.

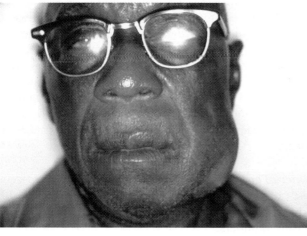

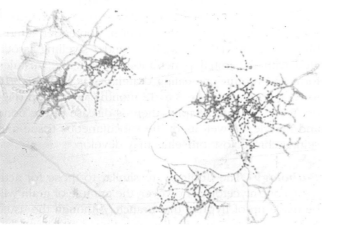

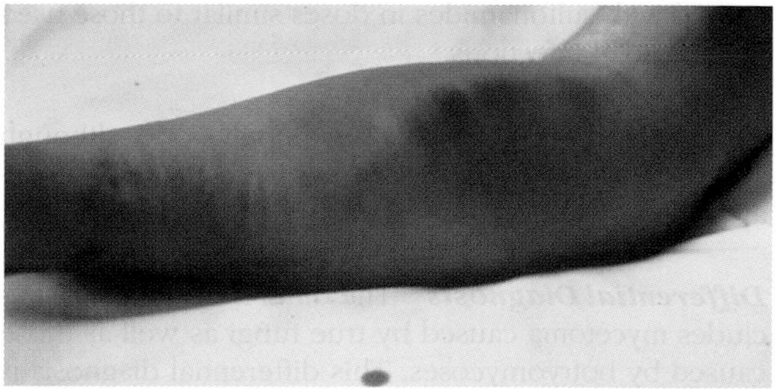

Figure 5.4 Nocardiosis presenting with a sporotrichoid spread. (Courtesy of Dr. Nancy Warren. From Elewski BE [ed]: Subcutaneous Fungal Infection. Blackwell Science, Cambridge, MA, with permission.)

Figure 5.3 Smear of *Nocardia* species stained with acid-fast stain. *Nocardia* species are partially acid-fast.

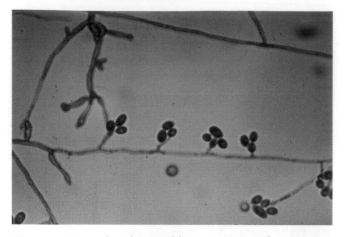

Figure 5.9 Lactophenol cotton blue preparation of *P. boydii*—the sexual phase of *Scedosporium apiospermum*.

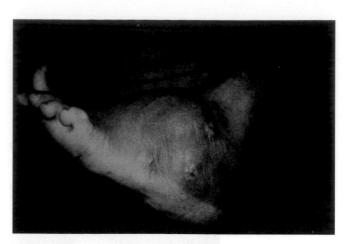

Figure 5.10 Eumycotic mycetoma on a foot.

Figure 5.12 Mycetoma of one foot due to *Actinomadura madurae*. (Courtesy of Dr. Nancy Warren.)

Figure 5.11 Mycetoma. (Courtesy of Dr. George Elgart, Department of Dermatology and Cutaneous Surgery, University of Miami.)

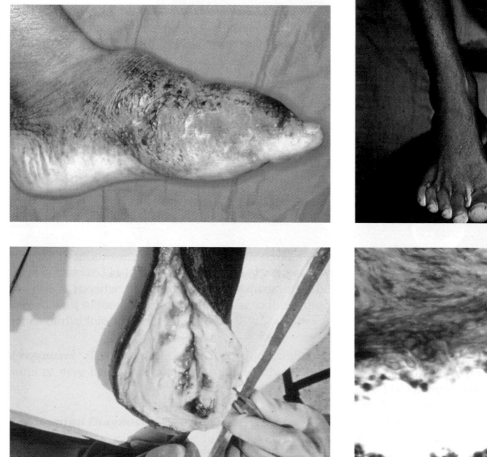

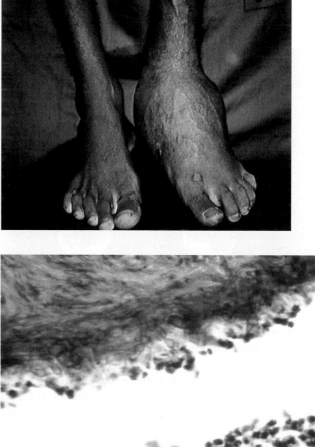

Figure 5.13 Mycetoma dissected open to show fibrosis and granules. (Courtesy of Dr. Nancy Warren. From Elewski BE [ed]: Subcutaneous Fungal Infection. Blackwell Science, Cambridge, MA, with permission.)

Figure 5.14 Edge of a eumycotic granule. (From Elewski BE [ed]: Subcutaneous Fungal Infection. Blackwell Science, Cambridge, MA, with permission.)

at the edge and as large as 12 μm. The fungi are periodic acid–Schiff (PAS)–positive and stain brown with Gomori's methenamine silver (GMS) stain.

Diagnosis Two factors are needed to make a diagnosis. First, the granule must be examined. On pathologic examination or even staining and direct examination of the granule, it shows the larger, swollen hyphae mentioned above. The difference in size allows one to distinguish between actinomycotic and eumycotic granules (Figure 5.15).

Another factor in diagnosis is culture. These granules may be planted on Sabouraud's dextrose agar, as well as on agar containing antibiotics. Slow growth should be seen over 2 to 4 weeks.

The organism most commonly cultured is *P. boydii* (the sexual form of *Scedosporium apiospermum*). These produce colonies that grow rapidly, becoming mousegray after beginning white. Some species characteristically have a ring of white around the edge. Microscopically, there are lemon-shaped annelloconidia, 4 to 9 to 6 to 19 μm, borne singly or in small groups[10] (Figs. 5.16 and 5.17). Although usually the cause of mycetoma, *P. boydii* has caused disseminated infection and death in the immunocompromised.

Other organisms that frequently may be isolated include *M. mycetomatis* and *M. grisea*. Both of these organisms produce a leathery colony that is slow growing and later develops aerial mycelia and diffusible pigment. The characteristics of these organisms are given in Table 5.2.

Treatment Early surgery is especially important in the treatment of eumycotic mycetomas.[11] However, amputation and radical surgery should be avoided. Instead, combination with medical management seems to work best.

Treatment with oral itraconazole is variable. Hay et al.[12] report that this drug produced improvement in 42% and no response in 33%. Welsh[13] reports success after ketoconazole failure. Ketoconazole long-term seems to show a higher rate of response but is ineffective in *P. boydii* infections.[1] Studies using terbinafine have not been reported.

Prognosis Without treatment, these infections are slowly progressive, producing first soft tissue injury, then bone damage. In severe cases, only surgical amputation has been necessary.

Differential Diagnosis The differential diagnosis includes mycetoma caused by actinomycetes as well as those caused by botryomycoses. This differential diagnosis is made by examining the granule microscopically. Other tumors can mimic the swelling, but not usually the draining sinuses and grains.

Botryomycotic Mycetoma

Etiology Botryomycosis is usually caused by organisms that, under other circumstances, cause disease that has a different appearance—cellulitis, abscess, and so on. Exactly what causes the formation of granules containing these bacterial organisms is not clear. The immune system and the method of inoculation of the organism are probably factors. Most patients with botryomycosis are obese, diabetics, alcoholics, or pa-

Table 5.2 Characteristics of Some of the Organisms that Cause Eumycotic Mycetoma

ORGANISM	COLONY	MICROSCOPIC	GRANULES
Acremonium species	Slow growing, cottony, white or buff	Crescent-shaped conidia in phialides at tips of conidiophores	White, soft, and small
Curvularia species	Dematiaceous	Three to five celled conidia with a swollen central cell	Dark, spherical, in animals
Leptosphaeria senegalensis	Rapid growing gray-brown	Elongated ascospores	Black, soft
Madurella grisea	Dark, leathery and folded	Occasional chlamydospores	Black, hard
Madurella mycetomatis	Leathery, heaped, folded, brown	Flask shaped phialides produce round conidia	Black, "open" or clear center, and small
Pseudallescheria boydii	Rapid growth, white and fluffy, becoming gray	Large, pyriform annelloconidia, borne singly, or in small groups	White, soft, and large

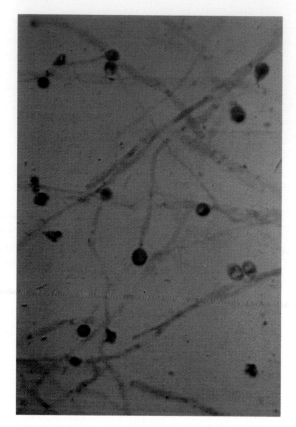

Figure 5.16 Microscopic view of a *Scedosporium apiospermum.*

Figure 5.15 Close-up view of a eumycotic granule.

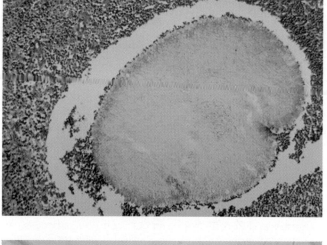

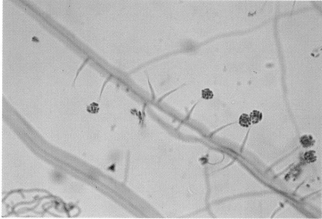

Figure 5.17 Lactophenol cotton blue preparation of *Acremonium* species, the second most common cause of eumycotic mycetoma.

tients showing general disability. Injection of mice with *Pseudomonas aeruginosa* and an adjuvant was able to reproduce the disease.[14]

Geographic Distribution The bacteria that cause botryomycosis have a worldwide distribution. The disease is rare.

Clinical Features Patients show disease similar to actinomycosis and mycetoma. Botryomycosis is part of the differential diagnosis of any disease with draining sinuses and grains.

Pathology Changes are identical to those of eumycotic mycetoma except for the granules or grains, which are described below.

Diagnosis The diagnosis of botryomycosis depends on isolation of the granule or grain and examination microscopically. These grains, unlike those of actinomycotic mycetoma or eumycotic mycetoma, are made up of clumps of bacteria and no filaments (Fig. 5.18). Gram-negative as well as gram-positive bacteria may be seen. Culture will be helpful. The following organisms have been reported to have produced this disease: *Staphylococcus aureus, Staphylococcus epidermidis, P. aeruginosa, Escherichia coli, Bacteroides* species, *Proteus* species, and *Streptococcus* species.

Treatment Treatment depends on the organism isolated. Because adequate tissue levels may be important, high doses and prolonged treatment may be necessary. In some instances, rapid resolution has been documented.[15] In addition, correction of the obesity or other disability may be of value.

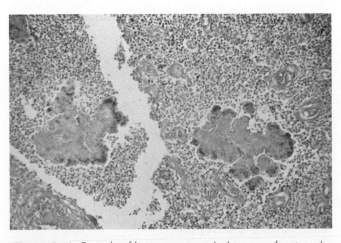

Figure 5.18 Granule of botryomycosis. At this magnification, the etiology of the granule is difficult to establish. (Courtesy of Dr. Nancy Warren.)

Prognosis Usually, there is a slow response to antibiotics.

Differential Diagnosis Any of the "mycetoma" diseases have the other diseases as part of the differential diagnosis. Examination of the grain and culture are necessary for adequate differentiation.

CHROMOBLASTOMYCOSIS

Etiology

Chromoblastomycosis is an infection caused by a group of fungi that produce darkly pigmented hyphae on media but produce Medlar bodies (sclerotic bodies, copper pennies) in tissue. These do not bud but produce new cells by forming a wall within the single-celled organism. The word *blast* signifies budding, so the term *chromoblastomycosis* is theoretically incorrect. For that reason, some authors prefer the term *chromomycosis*. Others feel that the word *chromomycosis* is no different in meaning than *phaeohyphomycosis* and cannot distinguish the fungi that produce chromoblastomycosis from those darkly pigmented fungi that produce disease as opportunists. McGinnis[16] prefers the term *chromoblastomycosis,* even though mycologically incorrect, for this disease and *phaeohyphomycosis* for opportunistic disease in which pigmented hyphae cause disease.

The disease was first described by Pedroso in Brazil in 1911, although the case was not published until 1920. The first published report was by Lane and Medlar in the United States. Dr. Medlar's subsequent description of the fungus led to his name being applied to the sclerotic bodies.

Geographic Distribution

Chromoblastomycosis is a disease of barefoot agricultural workers, mainly male. The organisms have been found in soil and in decaying wood. It is seen in all parts of the world but has a predilection for subtropical and tropical areas.

Clinical Features

The disease most often begins with the implantation of fungal elements into a foot. A verrucous granuloma is produced, usually on one leg (Fig. 5.19). The infection has some of the clinical and microscopic appearance of blastomycosis—warty edge with central clearing, transepidermal elimination of fungi, no obvious systemic disease, and pseudoepitheliomatous hyperplasia on microscopic examination—and its name derives from this similarity. The organisms that are seen, however, have pigment. An experimental disease mimicking the human condition has been described.[17]

As the fungus grows, there is a granulomatous response with pseudoepitheliomatous hyperplasia, producing verrucous areas on a single leg, with skip areas in between.[18] Bleeding and friability are obvious. Pustules are noted, as the organisms are eliminated across the epidermis. In this transepidermal elimination, organisms can be demonstrated in the pus as rounded, pigmented Medlar bodies. Scarring is often present in the center of lesions (Fig. 5.20).

Pathology

Biopsy shows a suppurative (i.e., containing neutrophils) granulomatous process with pseudoepitheliomatous hyperplasia and excess keratin production. Within the dermis, pigmented round bodies may be seen. These Medlar bodies represent the causative organism and are easily visualized without special stains[19] (Fig. 5.21).

Diagnosis

Diagnosis depends on demonstration of the causative organism. Five organisms produce this identical clinical picture. It is important to distinguish the organisms, since there are different responses to treatment among the several causes.

The organisms may be cultured on routine mycologic media, such as Sabouraud dextrose agar or mycosel agar. Colonies are black and slow growing. At first they appear to be a black yeasts, then later show hyphae on the surface. They are differentiated on the basis of sporulation. Three types of sporulation are present. In *Cladosporium* organisms, there are long, branching chains of conidia (Fig. 5.22). In *Phialophora* organisms, there is a vase-like structure (phial) containing the conidia (Fig. 5.23). In the *Rhinocladiella* (previously know as the *Acrotheca*) species, conidia are seen on a specialized conidiophore (Fig. 5.24). *Fonsecaea* species contain all three types of sporulation (Table 5.3). Other organisms have rarely been reported.[20]

Treatment

Itraconazole has been shown to be the most effective therapy. At a dose of 200 mg/day, there were no side effects, and 9 of 10 chronic patients had improvement.[21,22]

In cases caused by *Fonsecaea pedrosoi*, 5-fluorocytosine may be used in combination with the itraconazole. Sapercomazole, a newer imidazole not yet approved for use in the United States, has also been effective, in doses of 100 to 200 mg/day.[23]

Prognosis

Without treatment, the disease is progressive. Secondary bacterial infection has been seen, and late-onset squamous cell carcinoma has been seen in the scarred areas.

Differential Diagnosis

The differential diagnosis includes blastomycosis because of the similarity of presentation. However, blastomycosis presents in many areas other than the foot. In addition, the causative organism will be different.

Madura foot occurs in the same anatomic region but is clinically distinct because of the grains and draining sinuses.

SPOROTRICHOSIS

Etiology

The etiologic agent is *Sporothrix schenckii* found in decaying vegetation. Outbreaks have been found where there is trauma from wood or other vegetation and where there is sufficient humidity to support growth of the organism. The largest outbreak was in the gold mines of South Africa. In these mines, the humidity was high, and the roofs were supported by wooden struts. The organism grew on the wood and injured the workers. Over 2,000 cases were seen. The largest American epidemic was due to growth in sphagnum moss, with 84 cases in 15 states.[24,25]

The organism can exist worldwide, and the disease has been described sporadically on every continent. It is an occupational hazard among farmers, forestry workers, and horticulturists.

In addition to the usual transmission from decaying vegetation, transmission from a cat to a veterinarian has been reported.[26] Laboratory-acquired disease has been reported 10 times.[27]

Clinical Features

There are several patterns of presentation of cutaneous sporotrichosis. The usual pattern in an individual who has not previously been exposed is a lymphangitic

Figure 5.20 Chromoblastomycosis in Central America.

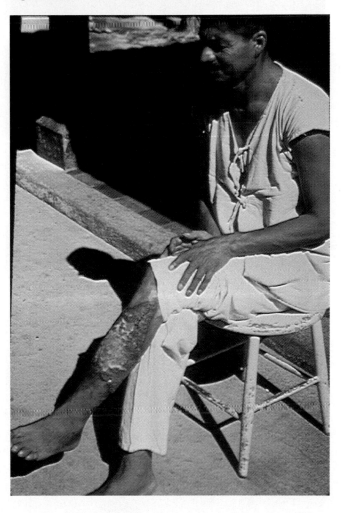

Figure 5.19 Chromoblastomycosis. (From Elewski BE [ed]: Subcutaneous Fungal Infection. Blackwell Science, Cambridge, MA, with permission.)

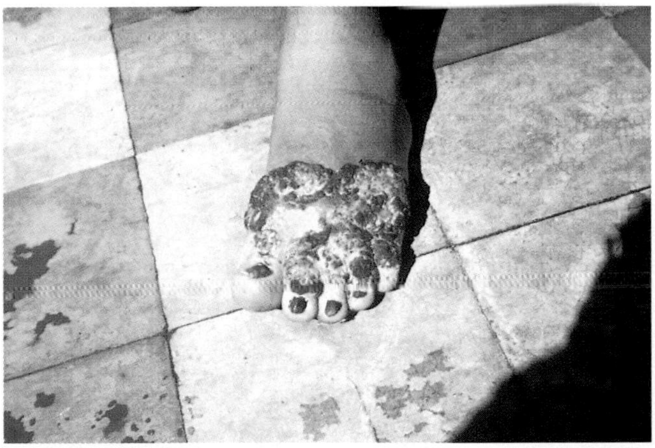

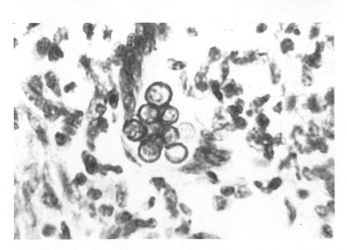

Figure 5.21 Chromoblastomycosis. Copper pennies (Medlar bodies) in tissue.

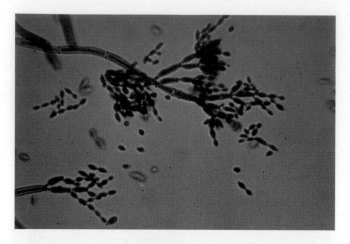

Figure 5.22 Microscopic view of *Cladosporium* species conidia formation.

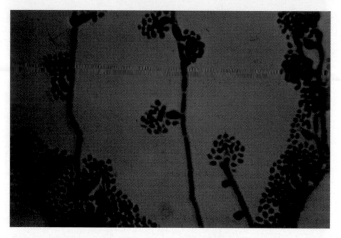

Figure 5.23 Microscopic view of *Phialophora* species conidia formation.

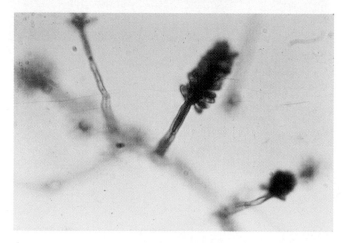

Figure 5.24 Microscopic view of *Rhinocladiella* species conidia formation.

Table 5.3 Conidia Formation in Organisms that Cause Chromoblastomycosis

ORGANISM	PHIALOPHORA CONIDIA FORMATION	CLADOSPORIUM CONIDIA FORMATION	RHINOCLADIELLA CONIDIA FORMATION
Phialophora verrucosa	+ + +	−	−
Cladosporium carrionii	−	+ + +	−
Rhinocladiella (Acrotheca) aquaspersa	−	−	+ + +
Fonsecaea pedrosoi	+ +	+	+ to + +
Fonsecaea compacta	+ + (compact)	+	+ to + +

Abbreviations: + + +, heavy; + +, moderate; +, light; −, absent.

spread. This is so characteristic that it may be known as a "sporotrichoid" spread. There is an initial break in the skin, in which an organism is introduced, and then other lesions appear in a proximal pattern of nodules, some of them breaking down, along the lymphatics. The draining node may become involved, although this is rare (Fig. 5.25). The arm is the usual site, although the face may become involved in children (Figs. 5.26 and 5.27).

A second pattern is seen in patients previously exposed to the organism. These patients develop a single ulcer. There is no evidence of lymphangitic spread, and the pattern is known as "fixed" cutaneous sporotrichosis[28] (Fig. 5.28). On biopsy, the lesion shows a suppurative granuloma, and no organisms are seen.[29] There is a long list of differential diagnostic possibilities (see below).

A third pattern has been seen with multiple primary lesions. This is seen when several injuries occur at close to the same time, as when one is working with wood that has harbored the growth of the organism. Here, several lesions occur at the same time, all with eroded epidermis and little movement. Again, the differential diagnosis list is long. This pattern has been seen in the United States in patients fixing up old houses.[30]

Finally, there are cases of diffuse dissemination and of pulmonary sporotrichosis. These are rare and seem to occur in immunocompromised individuals.[31] In one report, an immunocompromised individual acquired a cutaneous abscess while handling the organism in the laboratory and without obvious trauma to the skin. Such reports underlie the necessity of treating these organisms with great care.[27] Joint disease and tenosynovitis have both been reported, although they are quite rare.[32]

Pathology

In the usual presentation, the biopsy shows a nonspecific, suppurative granuloma. Diagnosis is difficult to make from a biopsy unless one is lucky enough to see an asteroid body in tissue. Although written about in many texts, it is rarely seen. Otherwise, PAS and Gomori's methenamine silver stains are usually negative. When the patient is immunocompromised, cigar-shaped, multiple budding yeast organisms may be seen.

Diagnosis

The only way to make a diagnosis is by taking part of the biopsy material and sending it to the mycology laboratory for culture.

Cultures of *S. schenckii* on Sabouraud's dextrose agar at room temperature are at first white and leathery with growth in 3 to 5 days (Fig. 5.30). Later, hyphae appear at the surface, and they become mouse-gray and sometimes black. The microscopic appearance at room temperature is that of mold, with very fine conidiophores suspending the conidia near the hyphae (Fig. 5.31). Larger hyphae have occasionally been visualized, but they give rise to the more frequent smaller hyphae.[33]

The yeast form may be isolated using specially enriched media at body temperature. The organism shows cigar-shaped budding forms 5 to 7 μm in diameter (Fig. 5.32). The change from one form to another (yeast to mold and the reverse) should be seen to establish a diagnosis.

Text continued on page 83

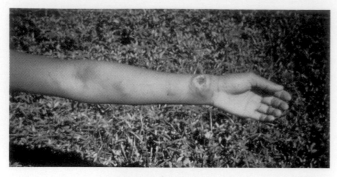

Figure 5.25 Sporotrichosis producing a lymphangitic spread on an arm.

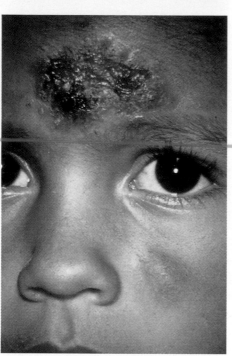

Figure 5.26 Sporotrichosis producing a lymphangitic spread on the face of a child.

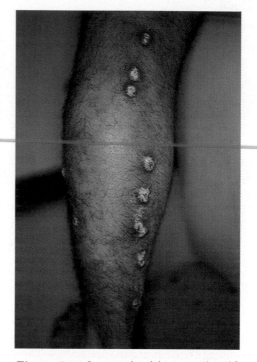

Figure 5.27 Sporotrichoid lesions. The differential diagnosis includes nocardiosis, sporotrichosis, swimming pool granuloma, leishmaniasis, and primary inoculation blastomycosis or coccidioidomycosis. In this case, the lesions represented nodular prurigo.

Figure 5.28 Sporotrichosis on the face. (Courtesy of Dr. Nancy Warren.)

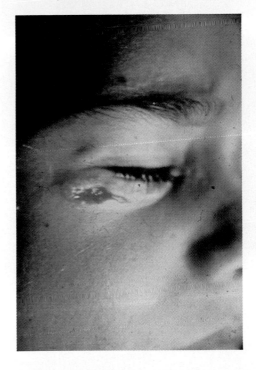

Figure 5.29 Sporotrichosis producing a solitary lesion: fixed cutaneous sporotrichosis.

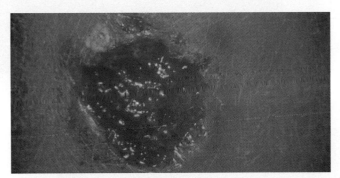

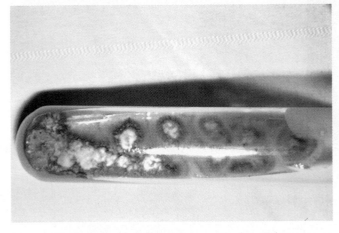

Figure 5.30 Culture of *Sporothrix schenckii*. Culture grows rapidly and is at first white, then mouse-gray.

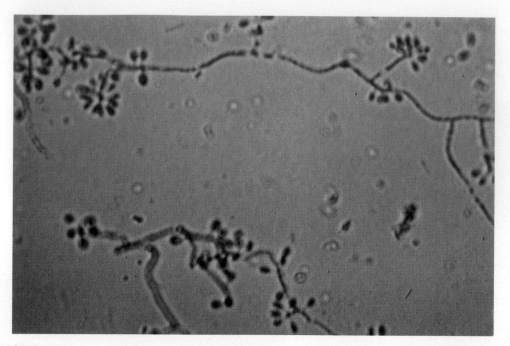

Figure 5.31 Sporotrichosis at room temperature, showing delicate conidiophores and conidia.

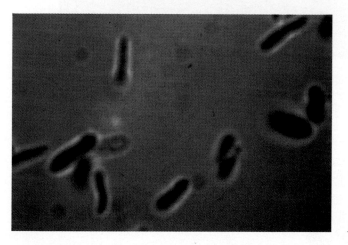

Figure 5.32 Sporotrichosis at 37°C showing cigar-shaped yeast

Table 5.4 General Overview of the Subcutaneous Mycoses

DISEASE	ORGANISM	TREATMENT
Actinomycotic mycetoma	*Actinomyces israelii*	Penicillin
Actinomycotic mycetoma	*Nocardia* species	Sulfonamides
Actinomycotic mycetoma	*Actinomadura* species	Sulfonamides and other broad-spectrum drugs
	Streptomyces species	
Eumycotic mycetoma	*Pseudallescheria boydii* and others	Itraconazole, surgery
Botryomycotic mycetoma	Bacteria	Antibiotics
Sporotrichosis	*Sporothrix schenckii*	Itraconazole, terbinafine
Chromoblastomycosis	*Cladosporium carrionii Fonsecaea* species	Itraconazole alone or with 5-fluorocytosine
	Phialophora verrucosa	
	Rhinocladiella aquaspersa	

Treatment

Saturated solution of potassium iodide (SSKI) is effective. The mode of action is unclear, since the organisms can grow easily in the presence of SSKI. Nevertheless, iodides are used with some efficacy, although the taste is bad, and some physicians are concerned about the effect on the thyroid.[34]

Itraconazole in doses of 200 mg/day seems to be a safe and dependable way to deal with this disease. In series of 30 cases in 27 patients, there were cures in 25 at doses of 200 to 400 mg/day.[35]

Similarly, terbinafine has shown promise. In one series, five cases responded to 250 mg twice daily, with negative cultures in 3 to 8 weeks, one in 12 weeks, and one in 32 weeks.[36]

Prognosis

The prognosis is good, even without treatment in immunocompetent individuals. Spontaneous healing has been reported.[37] However, pulmonary or disseminated disease may produce progressive disease with death.

Differential Diagnosis

Several infections can produce a lymphangitic spread. The most frequent offenders are the "MOTT" (mycobacteria other than tuberculosis) organisms. *Mycobacterium marinum,* when introduced while cleaning a fish tank, can produce the identical picture. Leishmaniasis (also known as pian bois), especially prevalent in South America, may have a similar appearance. Indeed, many primary inoculation diseases, particularly laboratory accidents causing disease from blastomycosis, histoplasmosis, or coccidioidomycosis, may produce a similar picture.

The differential diagnosis in fixed cutaneous sporotrichosis is more complicated (Fig. 5.27). Here, we have an ulcer, with no obvious changes, and a granulomatous histology. Tuberculosis, other fungal infections, leishmaniasis (especially leishmaniasis recidivans), sarcoidosis, foreign body reaction, and even cancer may be considered. Further biopsies with cultures are needed to determine the cause. Since the organism cannot be easily visualized, culture is the definitive test.

CONCLUSION

Table 5.4 summarizes the causative organisms and treatments of the subcutaneous mycoses.

REFERENCES

1. McGinnis M: Mycetoma. Dermatol Clin 14:97, 1996

2. Lopez Martinez R, Mendez Tovar LJ, Lavalle P et al: Epidemiology of mycetoma in Mexico: study of 2105 cases. Gac Med Mex 128:477, 1992

3. Lerner PI: The lumpy jaw: cervicofacial actinomycosis. Infect Dis Clin North Am 2:203, 1988

4. Warren N: Actinomycosis, nocardiosis, and actinomycetoma. Dermatol Clin 14:85, 1996

5. Zlotnik H, Buckley HR: Experimental production of actinomycetoma in BALB/c mice. Infect Immun 29:1141, 1980

6. Elgart ML: Subcutaneous mycoses. p. 155. In Elewski BE (ed): Cutaneous Fungal Infections. Igaku-Shoin, New York, 1992

7. Castro LG, Belda Junior W, Salebian A, Cuce LC: Mycetoma: a retrospective study of 41 cases seen in Sao Paulo, Brazil, from 1978 to 1989. Mycoses 36:89, 1993

8. Magana M, Magana GM: Mycetoma. Dermatol Clin 7:203, 1989

9. Malekzadeh M, Overturf GD, Auerbach SB, Wong L, Hirsch M: Chronic, recurrent osteomyelitis caused by *Scedosporium inflatum.* Pediatr Infect Dis J 9:357, 1990

10. Rippon JW: Medical Mycology. WB Saunders, Philadelphia, 1998

11. Fahal AH, Hassan MA: Mycetoma. Br J Surg 79:1138, 1992

12. Hay RJ, Mahgoub ES, Leon G, al Sogair S, Welsh O: Mycetoma. J Vet Med Mycol 30, suppl. 1:41, 1992

13. Welsh O: Mycetoma: current concepts in treatment. Int J Dermatol 30:387, 1991

14. Mackinnon JE, Conti-Diaz IA, Gezuele E et al: Experimental botryomycosis produced by *Pseudomonas aeruginosa.* J Med Microbiol 3:369, 1969

15. Findlay GH, Vismer HF: Botryomycosis: some African cases. Int J Dermatol 29:340, 1990

16. McGinnis MR: Chromoblastomycosis and phaeohyphomycosis: new concepts, diagnosis, and mycology. J Am Acad Dermatol 8:1, 1983

17. Ahrens J, Graybill JR, Abishawl A, Tio FO, Rinaldi MG: Experimental murine chromomycosis mimicking chronic progressive human disease. Am J Trop Med Hyg 40:651, 1989

18. Elgart G: Chromoblastomycosis Dermatol Clin 14:17, 1996

19. Uribe F, Zuluaga AI, Leon W, Restrepo A: Histopathology of chromoblastomycosis. Mycopathologica 105:1, 1989

20. Barba Gomez JF, Mayorga J, McGinnis MR, Gonzalez Mendoza A: Chromoblastomycosis caused by *Exophiala spinifera*. J Am Acad Dermatol 26:367, 1992

21. Restrepo A, Gonzalez A, Gomez I, Arango M, de Bedout C: Treatment of chromoblastomycosis with itraconazole. Ann NY Acad Sci 544:504, 1988

22. Kumar B, Kaur I, Chakrabarti A, Sharma VK: Treatment of deep mycoses with itraconazole. Mycopathologica 115:169, 1991

23. Franco L, Gomez I, Restrepo A: Saperconazole in the treatment of systemic and subcutaneous mycoses. Int J Dermatol 31:725, 1992

24. Dixon M, Salkin F, Duncan R et al: Isolation and characterization of *Sporothrix schenckii* from clinical and environmental sources associated with the largest U.S. epidemic of sporotrichosis. J Clin Microbiol 29:1106, 1991

25. Coles FB, Schuchat A, Hibbs JR et al: A multistate outbreak of sporotrichosis associated with sphagnum moss. Am J Epidemiol 136:475, 1992

26. Reed KD, Moore FM, Geiger GE, Stemper ME: Zoonotic transmission of sporotrichosis: case report and review [see comments]. Clin Infect Dis 16:384, 1993

27. Cooper CR, Dixon DM, Salkin IF: Laboratory-acquired sporotrichosis. J Vet Med Mycol 30:169, 1992

28. Sperling LC, Read SI: Localized cutaneous sporotrichosis. Int J Dermatol 22:525, 1984

29. Bickley LK, Berman IJ, Hood AF: Fixed cutaneous sporotrichosis: unusual histopathology following intralesional corticosteroid administration. J Am Acad Dermatol 12:1007, 1985

30. Yalisove BL, Berzin M, Williams CM: Multiple pruritic purple plaques: cutaneous sporotrichosis. Arch Dermatol 127:721, 1991

31. Callen JP, Kingman J: Disseminated cutaneous *Nocardia brasiliensis* infection. Pediatr Dermatol 2:49, 1984

32. Hay EL, Collawn SS, Middleton FG: *Sporothrix schenckii* tenosynovitis: a case report. J Hand Surg 11:431, 1986

33. Shadomy HJ, Wang H: Unusual structures of *Sporothrix schenckii*. Mycopathologica 102:143, 1900

34. Lesher JL, Jr, Fitch MH, Dunlap DB: Subclinical hypothyroidism during potassium iodide therapy for lymphocutaneous sporotrichosis. Cutis 53:128, 1994

35. Sharkey Mathis PK, Kauffman CA, Graybill JR et al: Treatment of sporotrichosis with itraconazole: NIAID Mycoses Study Group. Am J Med 95:279, 1993

36. Hull PR, Vismer HF: Treatment of cutaneous sporotrichosis with terbinafine. Br J Dermatol 126, suppl. 39:51, 1992

37. Bargman H: Sporotrichosis of the skin with spontaneous cure: Report of a second case [letter]. J Am Acad Dermatol 8:261, 1983

CHAPTER 6

Management and Therapy for Cutaneous Fungal Infection

Piet De Doncker

Gerald E. Piérard

SUMMARY

Diagnosis Examination of skin scrapings in KOH solution is routine and effective in demonstrating dermatophytes; cultures are required to make a definitive diagnosis

Topical Treatment of Superficial Cutaneous Mycoses Infection by dermatophytes, infection by *Candida* species, infection by *Malassezia* species, galenic forms of antifungals

Systemic Treatment Griseofulvin, ketoconazole, fluconazole, itraconazole, terbinafine

General Considerations for the Management of Superficial Infections Tinea infections (tinea corporis, tinea cruris, tinea pedis, tinea manus, tinea capitis, onychomycosis), cutaneous yeast infections (pityriasis versicolor, candidal infections), children

Recognition of fungal taxa is relevant with regard to epidemiologic concerns and risk of invasiveness. In human superficial infection, fungi adhere to and invade the stratum corneum, nails, and hair shafts, seldom penetrating living tissues. Thus, topical treatment has been recommended for superficial dermatophyte and yeast infections limited to the epidermis. Systemic agents are usually reserved for disease that is extensive, affects hair and nails, and is not responsive to topical agents. They are mandatory in deep-seated and invasive systemic mycoses.

There is an indispensable rule that if a cutaneous mycosis is suspected, the provisional diagnosis must be validated by demonstration of the pathogenic microorganism to ensure a successful treatment. Errors occur if the treatment is based on the clinical aspect alone. In clinical practice, two parameters must be considered in determining cure of a cutaneous mycosis: clinical cure and mycologic cure evaluated by both microscopy and culture. Total cure is achieved only when both of these parameters are met. This is the main objective for giving antifungal therapy. We review the topical and systemic treatment modalities that are available or being studied in different indications and prophylactic and other nonpharmacologic hygienic measures to overcome recurrences of fungal infections.

Predictive Evaluation of Antifungal Activity

In vitro testing and animal experiments are used to predict the activity of antifungals. In vitro data on the spectrum of activity depend on the conditions under which the tests are performed. Unfortunately, the tests available do not always identify the full pharmacologic profile of a drug. The correlation with the in vivo efficacy in human infection is not always adequate, particularly for N-substituted imidazole and triazole derivatives.[1] It is essential to design and use laboratory tests that most closely reflect the conditions of clinical practice. Comparative assessments on animals are time-consuming and only represent models without close correlation with fungal diseases in humans. Evaluations are even more difficult in the clinical situation where diseases are obviously heterogeneous with regard to the genera, species, and extent of infection and to the intervention of the natural host defenses against the infectious agent. Hence other predictive approaches have been designed for evaluating new compounds in the treatment of cutaneous mycotic diseases. An ex vivo method has been designed to evaluate more accurately the potential efficacy of antifungals, either topical or oral, in the human stratum corneum.[2–7] Drugs are tested in their proprietary formulations on cultures of pathogenic fungi growing on stratum corneum harvested from healthy human volunteers. Both the antifungal activity and lingering effect after stopping treatment can be evaluated. Unlike the in vitro models, the ex vivo method enables one to compare the relative efficacies of different antifungal regimens and the duration of antimycotic effects. For the oral route of administration, the ex vivo method accounts for drug absorption and whether the agent reaches the stratum corneum in therapeutic concentrations. A ranking of proprietary antifungals was launched according to clinically relevant criteria of fungitoxic activity.[5] In general, in vivo and ex vivo results indicate that none of the currently available antifungals show total fungicidal activity. The ex vivo studies using human stratum corneum are useful for carrying out dosage-finding studies and to quickly obtain information about therapeutic dosing.

TREATMENT

Topical Treatment of Superficial Cutaneous Mycoses

The management of most superficial cutaneous mycoses begins with topical treatments, which must prevent growth and invasion of the stratum corneum by the causal microorganism.

Infection by Dermatophytes When dermatophytosis is caused by an anthropophilic dermatophyte, the cutaneous lesion tends to be chronic, persistent and recalcitrant to therapy. In contrast, the infection by zoophilic and geophilic organisms may spontaneously resolve after a period of pronounced inflammation. Recurrence is caused partly by reinfection and by the failure to eradicate the primary infection. The presence of a reservoir, such as the nail, where the pathogen can survive for a long period in spite of active treatment may explain relapses after therapy cessation.

The early antidermatophyte drugs were benzoic acid combined with salicylic acid, undecylenic acid, and tolnaftate. Griseofulvin has been reported to be ineffective topically. A major breakthrough in efficacy came with the synthetic imidazole derivatives. These agents have a spectrum of activity affecting many different microorganisms.[5,8–10] Long-term experience with the topical imidazoles has confirmed their safety, clinical efficacy, and reliability in eradicating cutaneous dermatophyte infections. Other unrelated products such as ciclopirox olamine and haloprogin also show good antidermatophyte activity. New classes of potent antidermatophyte drugs are the morpholines, represented by amorolfine, and allylamine derivatives, including naftifine and terbinafine.[10–15]

Topical imidazoles and allylamines have high rates of clinical efficacy, with cure rates over 70%. However, the causative pathogens are not similarly affected by the various antifungals, which show some differences in their activity spectrum. The antifungal should be applied at least 2 cm beyond the visible advancing edge of the lesion. As a rule, the topical medication should be applied twice a day for a minimum of 2 weeks, although a 4-week therapy may be appropriate in athlete's foot. Unfortunately, the minimum treatment period has not been clearly established for all agents. When tinea shows visual resolution, treatment should be continued for at least 1 week after the lesion clears because inflammation may resolve before extinction of the fungus.

Tinea cruris and tinea pedis have a substantial recurrence rate. Counseling about nonpharmacologic prophylactic measures is important, while daily maintenance therapy during disease-free intervals is rarely recommended. Dusting the groin or foot area regularly with an absorbent medicated powder is useful.[16] Nonpharmacologic measures also have an important role both in clearing the lesions and minimizing recurrences. Patients should be advised to follow stringent hygiene rules and dry the area thoroughly with a towel.

When a mixed infection is present such as in athlete's foot, topical imidazole derivatives exhibit activity against the commonly implicated dermatophytes as well as against some yeasts, saprophytic molds, and gram-positive bacteria. However, gram-negative bacteria, which may be present in erosive lesions, will not respond to such treatment. Therefore, prior to the antifungal application, footbaths with an antiseptic (e.g., potassium permanganate, povidone-iodine, chlorhexidine, or chlorofene) can be recommended to control the bacterial contamination or superinfection.

Combination topical corticoid-antifungal mixtures are available, but some may need restrictions on length of therapy and location of application. Caution must be particularly exercised when using combination products that contain potent atrophogenic steroids. These combined treatments may do more harm than good in some chronic infections. The fact that the imidazoles and allylamines exert by themselves an anti-inflammatory effect may obviate the need for a steroid in most cases.

Infection by Candida Species Superficial *Candida* infections may be topically treated using genera-specific drugs such as nystatin and amphotericin B. They also benefit from many azoles, amorolfine, naftifine, and ciclopirox olamine.

Infection by Malassezia Species *Malassezia ovalis* is a member of the normal skin flora. It is associated with disease when the yeast form proliferates in excess and when the filamentous form (*Malassezia furfur*) develops. The yeast is sensitive to various topical agents including selenium sulfide, zinc pyrithione, and piroctone olamine. Among the current antifungal drugs, ketoconazole shows the highest anti-*Malassezia* effect.

Galenic Forms of Antifungals The use of topical antifungal drugs for superficial skin disease may be of limited success. Reasons explaining the clinical failures include lengthy treatment duration, poor patient compliance, and high relapse rates on some body sites. Because of these shortcomings, innovative formulations have been designed. Lotions, powders, shampoos, liposomal creams, and lacquers are among other special forms of drug delivery that have proven success in some clinical presentations.

Treatments for onychomycoses are numerous. Traditional methods have been limited by the lack of efficacy and difficulties in patient compliance. Topical therapy alone is sometimes effective when the disease is localized to the distal nails. However, in most cases, it is not successful in eradicating onychomycosis. Chemical, surgical, or laser avulsion of the thickened nail plate is an adjuvant procedure that may be indicated in combination with topical antifungals. It is possible to remove a nail without surgery by the use of ointments containing no less than 30% salicylic acid, 50% potassium iodide, or 40% urea. These preparations also improve the antifungal drug penetration, which can be enhanced still further by the use of occlusive dressings. Evolving topical therapy includes specific formulations for nails such as amorolfine, tioconazole and ciclopirox olamine lacquers, bifonazole-urea mixture, and butenafine gel.

Systemic Treatment

Oral antifungals are generally required for the treatment of chronic widespread or extensive skin infections as well as for hair and nail involvement. They are also used in patients who failed on topical therapy, in those with granulomatous lesions, and in immunosuppressed patients, by disease or drugs.

Griseofulvin and ketoconazole are losing ground in the treatment of dermatomycosis because of the duration of treatment, relatively low cure rates, and uncertainty about the safety profile. New and more effective oral therapies have marked a turning point in the treatment of cutaneous fungal infections, especially for onychomycosis. Pharmacokinetic studies have demonstrated the importance of the different excretion routes between these agents. For antifungal drugs whose main delivery route is via sebum, infections of palms and soles with their thick horny layer, abundance of sweat glands, and absence of sebaceous glands will respond differently than infections of the glabrous skin. For nails,

the way these agents penetrate into the nail unit and the persistence of drug levels in the nail unit have facilitated short treatment schedules with more recently the introduction of intermittent therapies.

All the antifungal agents show great diversity in their pharmacokinetic profiles and mechanism of actions. They may cause minor to moderate side effects. The decision of whether to treat by the topical or oral route is usually made on the basis of different factors, particularly the cure rate and the prevalence of unacceptable side effects (risk-benefit ratio). Optimum treatment of fungal infections depends on a thorough understanding of the differences in the spectrum of activity, pharmacology, and pharmacokinetics of antifungal drugs and how they affect the individual patient.

The ideal antifungal must be active against the causative organisms, penetrate infected tissues effectively, remain in these tissues in sufficient concentrations to produce an antifungal effect, have low retention in serum and other organs, and be safe. This combination of attributes permits short treatment regimens and minimizes side effects.

Griseofulvin Griseofulvin is produced by the metabolism of *Penicillium griseofulvum*.[17] Its spectrum is confined to dermatophytes. It inhibits nucleic acid synthesis and cell mitosis by arresting division at metaphase.[18] It may also limit the growth of dermatophytes by altering the sliding of microtubules necessary for the separation of chromosomes.[10]

The normal adult dose is 500 to 1,000 mg/day of microsize griseofulvin (MSG) or 250 to 500 mg of ultramicrosize griseofulvin (UMSG) to be given with fatty food, and the dosage for children is restricted to 10 mg/kg/day. Although a correlation between griseofulvin plasma concentrations and the clinical results was suggested, the microsize formulation did not prove to be better than the conventional griseofulvin.

Treatment should be continued until clinical and mycologic recovery (Fig. 6.1), which means 2 to 4 weeks for tinea corporis and tinea cruris, 4 to 8 weeks for tinea pedis and tinea manus, 6 to 8 weeks for tinea capitis, and for onychomycosis until complete replacement of infected tissue with healthy nail (5 to 6 months for fingernails, 8 to 18 months for toenails).[10,17,18] Although most griseofulvin therapy is conducted using daily doses, single megadoses of 3 to 5 g of griseofulvin have found support for the treatment of tinea capitis. Weekly treatment protocols have also been used successfully.

The best results with griseofulvin are obtained in the treatment of tinea capitis (due to *Microsporum canis*), tinea corporis, and tinea cruris. The cure rates of tinea capitis can be as high as 93%.[19] However, griseofulvin's activity is disappointing in onychomycosis, especially in

1. Continuous dosing of 500 mg - 1000 mg MSG or 250 - 500 mg UMSG daily

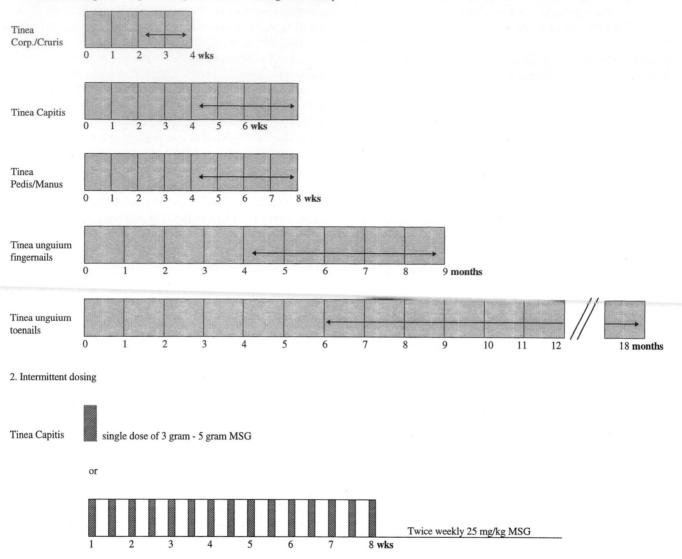

Figure 6.1 Treatment guidelines for griseofulvin in superficial dermatophytoses.

toenail disease.[20] Success of treatment in fingernails is expected to range between 50 and 60% and for toenails is not more than 20 to 30%. Besides the low cure rate, recurrences are frequent in toenails (±60%), and time to relapse can be as short as 3 months after stopping treatment.

In general, the drug is well tolerated.[18,20] The most common adverse events encountered are headache and gastrointestinal intolerance, and these may be reasons for discontinuing treatment. Less common adverse effects include urticaria and photosensitivity, hematologic effects including leukopenia, chronic anemia, and precipitation of a porphyria cutanea tarda in predisposed persons. Monthly hematologic examinations are advised as routine laboratory tests. Griseofulvin interacts with the metabolism of phenobarbital, primidone, anticoagu-

lants (coumarin derivatives), oral contraceptives, cyclosporine, alcohol, and some photosensitizing drugs.[18,20]

Ketoconazole Ketoconazole, the first imidazole exhibiting a broad-spectrum antifungal activity against most superficial fungal pathogens (dermatophytes, dimorphic fungi, yeasts) and some gram-positive bacteria,[18,21] inhibits the synthesis of ergosterol, the major sterol constituent of fungal cell walls, vital for cellular growth.[10,18]

The imidazole derivatives inhibit 14α-demethylase, a cytochrome P-450–dependent enzyme intervening in membrane ergosterol synthesis. The accumulation of lanosterol and the depletion of ergosterol following such inhibition are responsible for functional disorders of the membrane (increased membrane permeability) and disruption of the associated membrane enzymes, thus affecting the growth and viability of the fungal cell.[20] Oral ketoconazole interferes with several human cytochrome P-450 enzymes as well, and this aspect is clinically relevant for long-term use and use of higher dosages of the drug.[10]

Sweat is the most important delivery route by which ketoconazole reaches the skin, although the drug shows also strong keratin adherence. Inhibitory concentrations are maintained in the stratum corneum for at least 10 days after termination treatment.

The usual adult dosage is 200 mg/day with the main meal, which promotes absorption of the drug. It may be increased to 400 to 600 mg/day such as in chronic mucocutaneous candidiasis.[22]

Treatment is given until clinical and mycologic recovery (Fig. 6.2). This means ±4 weeks for tinea corporis or tinea cruris and 6 to 8 weeks for the plantar type of tinea pedis. A response rate of 94% is reported for tinea corporis and tinea cruris, with a median treatment length of 3 weeks; 77% for tinea pedis and tinea manus, with a median treatment length of 5 weeks; 89% for cutaneous candidiasis, with a median treatment length of 3 weeks; and 73% for tinea capitis, with a median treatment length of 8 weeks.[23] *M. canis* is a much more difficult organism to treat with ketoconazole for fungal infections of the scalp. For pityriasis versicolor, treatment duration is shorter, with a median duration of 2 weeks resulting in a 93% response (n = 468). Ketoconazole has also been used to treat *Malassezia*-induced folliculitis and seborrheic dermatitis.

In onychomycosis, a mean cure rate of 85% is reported for fingernail infections (range = 52 to 100%) and 74% for toenails (range = 19 to 100%), with an average duration of about 6.5 months (*Candida* infections) for fingernails and 7.5 to 12 months (dermatophyte infections) for toenail infections. Recurrences in toenail mycoses could reach 45%, although an average relapse rate of 12.5% is reported in all reviewed studies. Ketoconazole may certainly be considered for *Candida* onychomycosis, including chronic mucocutaneous candidiasis.

Intermittent regimens of ketoconazole (400 mg as a single bolus dose or repeated monthly) have been shown to be effective and safe for the treatment of tinea versicolor, and a once-weekly dose of 400 mg (repeated three to eight times) is also satisfactory in dermatomycosis (Fig. 6.2).

Ketoconazole is usually well tolerated, with an average incidence of minor side effects of 15% from all studies (range = 0 to 32.5%).[23] As a result of the possible side effects, interruption of treatment is sometimes necessary. Side effects include gastrointestinal intolerance,

nausea, and vomiting. In a review of 80 clinical studies, which collected data from 4,130 dermatologic patients treated with ketoconazole, the total prevalence of side effects was 7.7%, with the gastrointestinal adverse effects being the most frequently reported (4%).

Ketoconazole blocks human metabolic processes such as cytochrome P-450–dependent adrenal androgen biosynthesis, causing symptoms such as gynecomastia, impotence, oligo- and azoospermia, and decreased libido.[18,23] These effects are mainly seen at higher dose ranges (over 600 mg daily). An idiosyncratic form of drug-induced hepatitis has been associated with the drug. The risk of hepatitis has been assessed as 1 per 10,000 patients, and the effect is more frequent in patients with onychomycosis.[18,23] Onset of symptoms are usually observed after 2 months of treatment. Liver function tests should be performed twice monthly in the first 2 months and then once monthly.

Antacids, H_2 receptor antagonists (cimetidine, ranitidine, famotidine, nizatidine), and antisecretory agents (omeprazole) increase gastric pH, hence decreasing the absorption of ketoconazole. Ketoconazole is known to interact with coumarin derivatives, indanedione, cyclosporine, chlordiazepoxide, glucocorticoids, ethanol, insulin, terfenadine, astemizole, rifampicin, and phenytoin.[4,18,24]

Ketoconazole has presented an important turning point in the search for more effective drugs. Ketoconazole is mainly being used in superficial fungal infections, such as pityriasis versicolor and vaginal candidiasis, where the treatment duration is less than 2 weeks. Its use is not recommended for tinea unguium and tinea capitis due to *M. canis*. However, the widespread acceptance of its mechanism of action has created a revival of antimycotic research and widened the scope of pharmacologic possibilities with cytochrome P-450 blocking agents. Despite the fact that ketoconazole is used mostly for the treatment of fungal infections, this drug deserves to be viewed as a multiple-application compound. It inhibits thromboxane and leukotriene synthesis, inhibits the metabolism of retinoic acid, reduces androgen production, and secondly, may limit some effects of cytokines (like the acute inflammatory response mediators such as interleukin-1 and tumor necrosis factor α). The clinical possibilities of such a drug is still be evaluated.

Fluconazole Fluconazole is a water-soluble bis-triazole tertiary alcohol.[25] Initially, the drug was studied in systemic mycoses (histoplasmosis, coccidioidomycosis, cryptococcosis) and mucosal candidiasis.[9,25–27] Fluconazole was mainly used in acquired immunodeficiency syndrome (AIDS) and other immunocompromised patients.[26]

Figure 7.1 Histoplasmosis. Tuberculate macronidia of *Histoplasma capsulatum*. Culture at 37°C. Lactophenol with cotton blue stain.

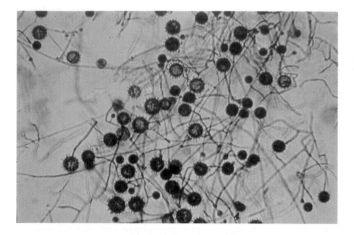

Figure 7.2 Bullous erythema multiforme associated with pulmonary histoplasmosis.

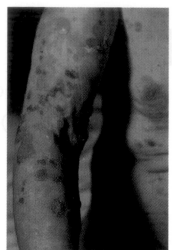

Figure 7.3 Disseminated histoplasmosis. Ulcer of the tongue. (Courtesy of Dr. Howard Larsh.)

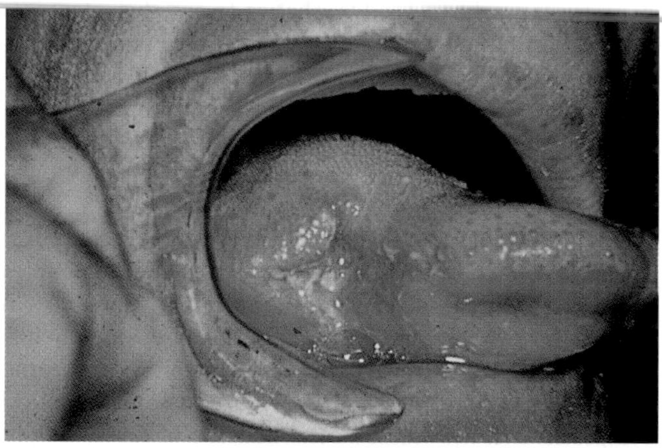

Figure 7.4 Disseminated histoplasmosis. Necrotic nodular lesion of the lip.

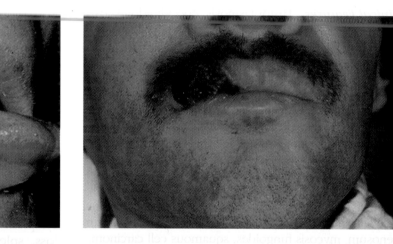

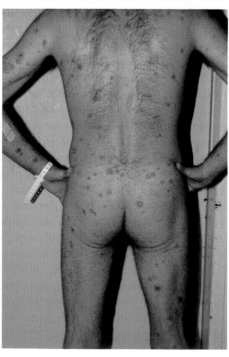

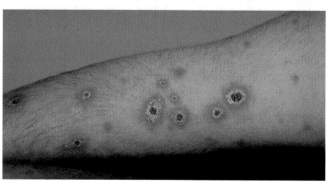

Figure 7.6 Disseminated histoplasmosis. Close-up of the lesions on the arm of the patient shown in Figure 7.5.

Figure 7.5 Disseminated histoplasmosis. Widespread necrotic papular eruption.

Pathology

A mixed dermal infiltrate is present, made up of neutrophils, lymphocytes, histiocytes, and giant cells. The organism appears in the cytoplasm of histiocytes and giant cells as numerous small spherical or oval yeast forms, 1 to 5 μm in diameter. They appear to be surrounded by a clear ring of space, a fixation artifact that resembles a capsule (Fig. 7.8). *H. capsulatum* is best demonstrated with the periodic acid–Schiff (PAS) stain.

Diagnosis

Asymptomatic pulmonary infections can be diagnosed retrospectively by skin test conversion and sometimes by characteristic patterns of calcification. Serologic tests, particularly the radioimmunoassay histoplasmin complement fixation tests, are useful in screening and monitoring progress. Demonstration of the organism in blood and bone marrow culture or buffy coat preparations, sputum, urine sediment, splenic puncture, or skin and mucous membrane biopsies provides the most reliable diagnostic evidence (Fig. 7.9).

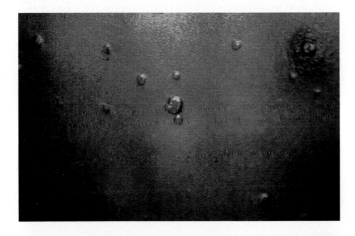

Figure 7.7 Disseminated histoplasmosis. Papular lesions resembling molluscum contagiosum. The patient has AIDS. (From Crissey J, Lang H, Parish L: Diseases caused by thermally dimorphic fungi. In Manual of Medical Mycology. Blackwell Science, Cambridge, MA, 1995, with permission.)

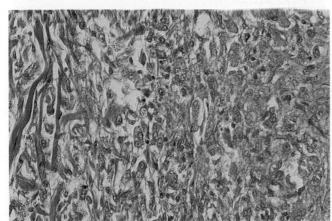

Figure 7.8 Histoplasmosis. Intracellular *Histoplasma capsulatum*. Skin biopsy, hematoxylin-eosin stain.

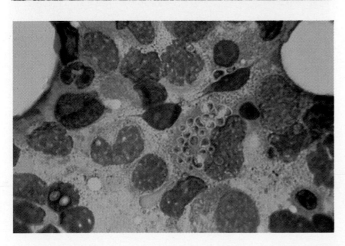

Figure 7.9 Histoplasmosis. *Histoplasma capsulatum*. Bone marrow, Wright's stain. (From Crissey J, Lang H, Parish L: Diseases caused by thermally dimorphic fungi. In Manual of Medical Mycology. Blackwell Science, Cambridge, MA, 1995, with permission.)

Treatment

Treatment is indicated only in the cavitary and disseminated forms of the disease. Itraconazole is the medication of choice in less severe forms of histoplasmosis. It is effective in more than 90% of cases. The recommended dosage is 300 mg PO bid for 3 days, followed by 200 mg PO bid for 3 to 12 months.

Amphotericin B is still recommended for initial treatment of life-threatening forms, particularly when the central nervous system is involved. It can be administered intravenously using peripheral veins or a central venous port. It is advisable to begin intravenous amphotericin B therapy with a 1-mg test dose before the first treatment dose is administered. This precaution is of some use in preventing acute hypersensitivity reactions but is of more value in identifying patients prone to the more severe adverse reactions of an acute nature that are related directly to the infusion of amphotericin B and occur in a significant number of patients. Included among these reactions are chills, fever, headache, nausea, and vomiting, usually beginning 2 to 3 hours after the start of the infusion. Infusion-related reactions may be less intense with subsequent doses. Ancillary medications useful in blunting infusion-related reactions include corticosteroids, meperidine, acetaminophen, and diphenhydramine.

The usual maintenance dose of amphotericin B is 0.5 to 1.0 mg/kg/day. This level is usually achieved by gradual incremental dose increases of 5 to 10 mg/day. Undue delay in reaching therapeutically effective levels may be detrimental to the patient. In patients with adequate renal function, amphotericin B can be infused 1 or 2 hours or longer (no more than 50 mg/h).

A total cumulative dose of 25 to 35 mg/kg is sufficient for most cases of histoplasmosis. Higher cumulative doses may be necessary for coccidioidomycosis. It is impossible to lay down hard and fast rules for total dose and treatment duration in many clinical situations. Disappearance or persistence of signs and symptoms, immune status, recoverability of the fungus, and the presence or absence of intercurrent disease are all factors to be taken into consideration in management of the individual case.

Nephrotoxic signs and symptoms are expected events in amphotericin B therapy, and nephrotoxicity is the major dose-limiting organ toxicity. Regular renal monitoring with correction of electrolyte imbalances is absolutely essential.

New formulations in which amphotericin B encapsulated into liposomes are less toxic and show great promise. They deliver higher blood levels, allowing a lower total dose.

Intrathecal use, recommended for central nervous system involvement, requires consultation with personnel specially trained in the technique.

Following an initial response to amphotericin B, itraconazole can be used for maintenance. Fluconazole is also under investigation as an alternative to amphotericin B.

All consenting patients with disseminated histoplasmosis should be tested for HIV infection. Suppressive treatment with itraconazole to prevent relapse is indicated in AIDS patients and should be continued indefinitely.[6,7]

The effectiveness and the optimum dosage and time schedules for treatment of this and other systemic mycoses with the newer antifungals have not yet been firmly established. Moreover, deleterious drug interactions have been observed with several of these medications. Clinicians are urged to consult the latest literature for guidance.

Differential Diagnosis

Miliary tuberculosis, lymphoma, and disseminated coccidioidomycosis, cryptococcosis, or penicilliosis (*Penicillium marneffei*) can be mimicked by histoplasmosis. Demonstration of the causative organism serves to establish the correct diagnosis.

COCCIDIOIDOMYCOSIS

Etiology

Coccidioidomycosis is caused by the thermally dimorphic fungus *Coccidioides immitis*. A soil saprophyte in its natural state, it enters the body by aerosol inhalation. Cultures at room temperature and 37°C are identical: fluffy grayish to brown colonies made up of mycelial elements that fragment easily and are dangerous to laboratory personnel (Fig. 7.10). Tissue forms are spherules

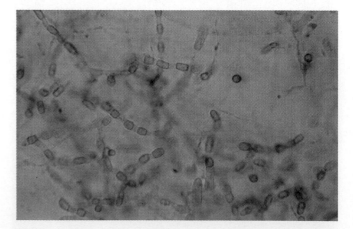

Figure 7.10 Coccidioidomycosis. *Coccidioides immitis*, culture at room temperature. Hyphae fragmenting into arthrospores that are easily dispersed and dangerous to laboratory personnel.

that fill with endospores and rupture. Endospores in turn become spherules, perpetuating the cycle.[2]

Clinical Features

Coccidioidomycosis is endemic in the drier areas of the southwestern United States and Mexico. Clinical forms include asymptomatic infections, self-limited pneumonia, chronic pulmonary disease, progressive pneumonia, extrapulmonary dissemination, and primary cutaneous inoculation.

Coccidioidomycosis begins as a pulmonary infection that is usually self-limited and asymptomatic; occasionally it presents with influenza-like symptoms. A few cases go on to develop a self-limited pneumonia, characterized by dry cough and pleuritic pain, and sometimes fever, night sweats, headache, and arthralgia. Healing usually takes place within 2 months. Erythema nodosum, erythema multiforme, or toxic erythema may be associated with any of these pulmonary infections (Fig. 7.11).

Extrapulmonary dissemination is uncommon. Endospores escape the lungs during initial infection to produce lesions at other sites. Filipino and black patients are most susceptible; it is more common in men, but pregnancy also predisposes. In endemic areas, dissemination often occurs as an opportunistic infection associated with AIDS.

Bone and joints are involved in some 50% of cases, particularly the spine, pelvis, hands, and lower extremities. Sinus tracts to the skin may develop. The most serious manifestation of dissemination is meningitis, which occurs in approximately one-third of the cases. If left untreated, it is fatal within 2 years. Gastrointestinal and genitourinary tract infections are also sometimes seen.

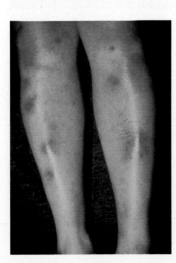

Figure 7.11 Coccidioidomycosis. Erythema nodosum associated with initial pulmonary infection.

Skin lesions occur early in some 40% of dissemination cases; the incidence later in the course is much higher. Papular lesions progress to nodules and plaques, often associated with pustules. Subcutaneous nodules, deep abscesses, cellulitis, and verrucous and fungating lesions may also be seen (Fig. 7.12 to 7.17). Scarring is often pronounced. No area is exempt, but the face, especially the nose and nasolabial folds, is the favored site. Extremities are also commonly involved.[2,5,8,9]

Primary cutaneous inoculation is rare. A pustule or nodule develops at the inoculation site, ulcerates, and is sometimes accompanied by lymphangitis and regional adenopathy (Fig. 7.18).

Pathology

Pseudoepitheliomatous hyperplasia is often present. Dermal reaction can range from acute and purulent to chronic inflammation and even granuloma formation. Organisms are usually present in significant numbers and in all stages of the spherule-endospore life cycle (Figs. 7.19 and 7.20). Mature spherules are large (diameter, 30 to 60 μm). Diameters of freshly extruded endospores average 5 μm. *C. immitis* is visible in hematoxylin-eosin–stained sections but is better visualized with the PAS stain (Fig. 7.20).

Diagnosis

Serologic agglutination and immunodiffusion test and conversion of a negative coccidioidin skin test to positive provide useful confirmatory information, but demonstration of the spherules and endospores of *C. immitis* is essential to the diagnosis. The organism can often be found on direct examination of pus and scrapings from skin lesions; it is more elusive in sputum and cerebrospinal fluid. Cultures from these sites are also of value. PAS-stained preparations of skin lesion biopsy material provide the surest route to the diagnosis.

Treatment

Acute pulmonary cases need no treatment. Severe primary infections, infections in high-risk ethnic groups or in immunocompromised individuals, and all cases of dissemination should be treated. Amphotericin B, administered intravenously, remains the medication of choice. (See the section on histoplasmosis for details on the administration of this antibiotic.) When meninges are involved, amphotericin B should be administered intrathecally as well. Because of its excellent penetration

Figure 7.12 Disseminated coccidioidomycosis. Erythematous nodular lesion of the nose.

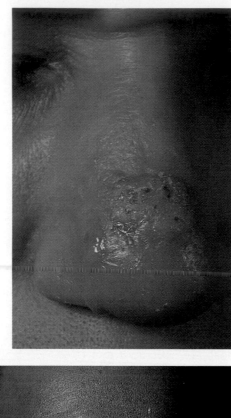

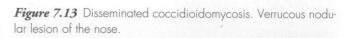
Figure 7.13 Disseminated coccidioidomycosis. Verrucous nodular lesion of the nose.

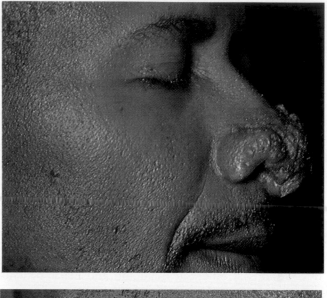

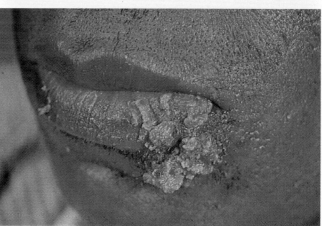

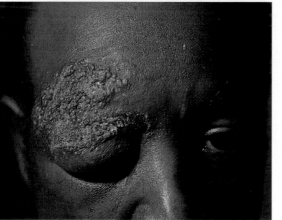

Figure 7.14 Disseminated coccidioidomycosis. Plaque lesion, left brow.

Figure 7.15 Disseminated coccidioidomycosis. Nodulopustular lesion, lower lip.

Figure 7.17 Disseminated coccidioidomycosis. Subcutaneous nodules, right supraclavicular area. (From Crissey J, Lang H, Parish L: Diseases caused by thermally dimorphic fungi. In Manual of Medical Mycology. Blackwell Science, Cambridge, MA, 1995, with permission.)

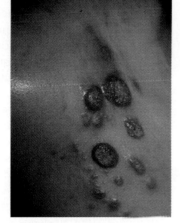

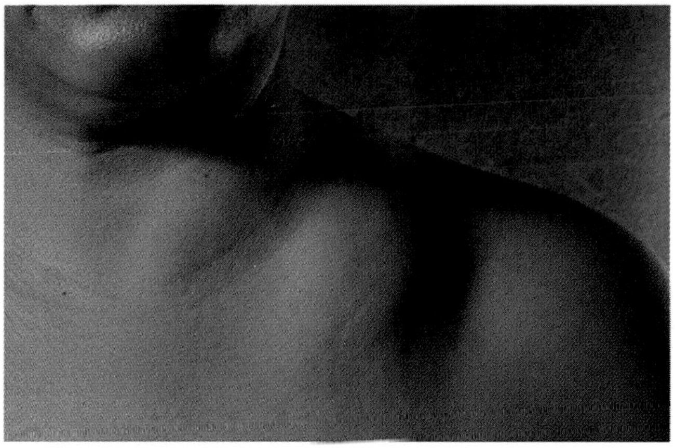

Figure 7.16 Disseminated coccidioidomycosis. Nodular lesions, anterior chest.

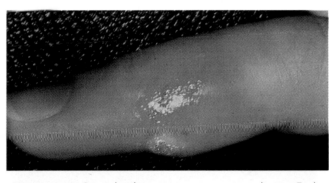

Figure 7.18 Coccidioidomycosis, primary inoculation. Erythematous pustular lesion, finger.

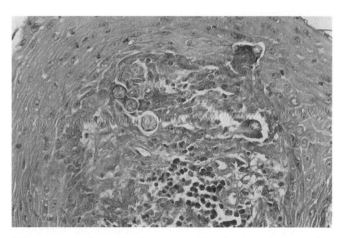

Figure 7.19 Coccidioidomycosis. Skin biopsy, hematoxylin-eosin stain.

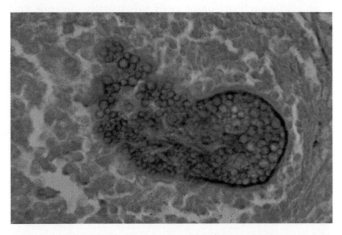

Figure 7.20 Coccidioidomycosis. Skin biopsy, PAS stain. *Coccidioides immitis*, mature spherule extruding endospores.

toxylin-eosin preparations often appear as round holes punched in the cytoplasm. Mother cells average 10 μm in diameter and reproduce with a single thick-necked bud (Fig. 7.27). Organisms are usually few in number and are best demonstrated with the PAS stain.

Diagnosis

Demonstration of *B. dermatitidis* in potassium hydroxide preparations of sputum and skin lesion scrapings provides the most convenient route to the diagnosis (Fig. 7.28). Pustules at the periphery of the skin lesions are particularly good places to look. The organism is identifiable in skin biopsy sections. Cultures of sputum and skin lesion material are also useful. Skin test and serologic test are not reliable.

Treatment

Because no reliable method exists to predict which patients will develop serious disease, it is recommended that all identified cases be treated. Blastomycosis usually occurs in individuals with no evident degree of immunocompromise. Nevertheless, the disease in its most aggressive forms is being reported with increasing frequency as an opportunistic infection in patients with immunodeficiency. All consenting patients with disseminated blastomycosis should be tested for HIV infection.

Itraconazole is the medication of choice in less severe infections. It is effective in more than 90% of cases. The recommended dosage is 200 to 400 mg/day PO for 3 to 12 months. Amphotericin B is still recommended for initial treatment of life-threatening forms, particularly when

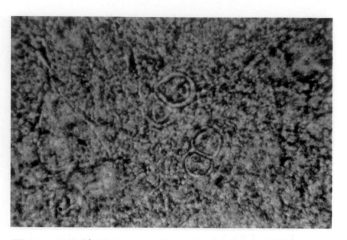

Figure 7.28 Blastomycosis. Potassium hydroxide preparation, sputum. *Blastomyces dermatitidis*, mother cells producing thick-necked single bands.

the central nervous system is involved. (See the section on histoplasmosis for details on the administration of this antibiotic.) Following an initial response to amphotericin B, itraconazole can be used for maintenance. Ketoconazole is an acceptable alternative.[5,11–13]

The effectiveness and the optimum dosage and time schedules for treatment of this and other systemic mycoses with the newer antifungals have not yet been firmly established. Moreover, deleterious drug interactions have been observed with several of these medications. Clinicians are urged to consult the latest literature for guidance.

Differential Diagnosis

Pyoderma gangrenosum, mycosis fungoides, squamous cell carcinoma, cutaneous tuberculosis, syphilitic gummata, and other deep mycoses can present with lesions indistinguishable clinically from cutaneous blastomycosis. Characteristic histopathology and demonstration of the organism will serve to establish the proper diagnosis.

PARACOCCIDIOIDOMYCOSIS

Etiology

Paracoccidioidomycosis is caused by the thermally dimorphic fungus *Paracoccidioides brasiliensis*. A soil saprophyte in its natural state, it enters the body by aerosol inhalation. When cultured at room temperature it appears as a wrinkled colony covered with a short nap of white mycelium and made up of mycelial elements

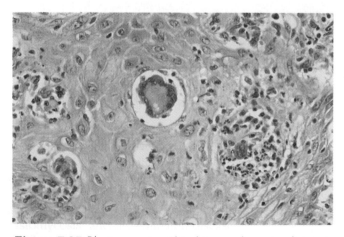

Figure 7.27 Blastomycosis. Skin biopsy, hematoxylin-eosin stain. *Blastomyces dermatitidis*, mother cell and thick-necked single buds.

bearing conidiophores, each of which supports a single conidium. At 37°C cultures are yeast-like and made up of mother cells bearing multiple buds, identical with the forms found in infected tissue (Fig. 7.29).[2,15]

Clinical Features

Paracoccidioidomycosis is limited to South and Central America, where it is the most common respiratory mycosis and a problem of major proportions. It is largely a disease of adults. Males outnumber females 15:1, the highest ratio for any mycosis.

The disease begins as an acute pneumonitis that may be asymptomatic and may abort or progress, with weight loss, weakness, anorexia, bloody purulent sputum, night sweats, and physical signs and radiologic findings suggesting lung abscess, carcinoma, or tuberculosis. The clinical picture often resembles pulmonary tuberculosis, with which it is frequently coexists.

Extrapulmonary dissemination is common and is usually associated with immunocompromise, induced in some instances by the fungus itself. Dissemination may occur months or years after the initial infection. It is increasingly observed as an opportunistic infection in AIDS patients. Untreated disseminated disease is uniformly fatal. Signs and symptoms are referable to the organ system involved. Spleen, lymph nodes, adrenal glands, intestines, liver, central nervous system, and bone may be affected.

Mucocutaneous lesions occur regularly. Erythematous areas appear on mucosal surfaces and ulcerate. Tongue, buccal mucosa, gingiva, lips, and palate may all be involved (Figs. 7.30 to 7.33). Dysphagia and voice change are common complaints. Teeth are lost, and eventually the patient is unable to eat. Skin is attacked initially by direct extension from mucosal lesions. Nodular, papillomatous, and frambesiform lesions may appear. Regional nodes become involved and break down to form draining fistulas. Hematogenous spread to distant skin sites often occurs, resulting in the formation of subcutaneous abscesses.[14-16]

Pathology

As in blastomycosis, pseudoepitheliomatous hyperplasia is prominent, sometimes with intraepidermal neutrophilic abscesses, along with a dense dermal infiltrate in which neutrophils predominate. Multinucleate giant cells are usually present and sometimes contain the organisms. Mother cells average 10 to 15 μm in diameter and reproduce with multiple buds to produce the pathognomonic "ship's wheel" configuration (Fig. 7.29).

This feature is not always evident, especially in sections stained with hematoxylin-eosin. Organisms are usually few in number; mother cells and buds are best demonstrated with PAS or silver stains (Fig. 7.34).

Diagnosis

Demonstration of the organism with its characteristic budding pattern by direct examination, biopsy, or culture will establish the diagnosis. Skin tests are unreliable. Serologic tests, particularly the agar gel immunodiffusion procedure, are useful for diagnostic confirmation.

Treatment

Itraconazole is the medication of choice. Ketoconazole is an acceptable alternative, fluconazole less so. Intravenous amphotericin B is recommended for advanced disseminated disease and for azole failures. (See the section on histoplasmosis for details on the administration of this antibiotic.) Sulfonamides are effective in some cases and are still used routinely in some parts of the world.[14-16]

The effectiveness and the optimum dosage and time schedules for treatment of this and other systemic mycoses with the newer antifungals have not yet been firmly established. Moreover, deleterious drug interactions have been observed with several of these medications. Clinicians are urged to consult the latest literature for guidance.

Differential Diagnosis

Squamous cell carcinoma, mucocutaneous tuberculosis, syphilitic gummata, and other deep mycoses, particularly histoplasmosis, can present with lesions indistinguishable clinically from paracoccidioidomycosis. Characteristic histopathology and demonstration of the organism will serve to establish the proper diagnosis.

PENICILLIOSIS (P. MARNEFFEI)

Etiology

P. marneffei, the cause of this form of penicilliosis, is the only dimorphic Penicillium organism. It is a natural pathogen of the bamboo rat indigenous to southeast Asia. Room temperature cultures on Sabouraud's

Figure 7.29 Paracoccidioidomycosis. Culture at 37°C. *Paracoccidioides brasiliensis*, mother cells bearing multiple buds, identical with the forms found in infected tissue.

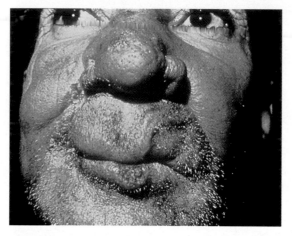

Figure 7.30 Paracoccidioidomycosis. Ulcerating nodular lesion, tongue.

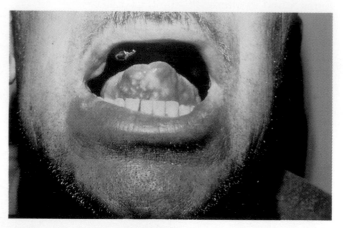

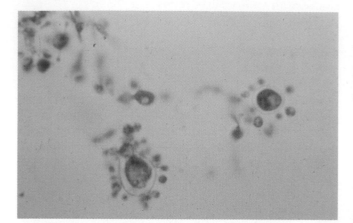

Figure 7.31 Paracoccidioidomycosis. Ulcerating nodular lesions, face.

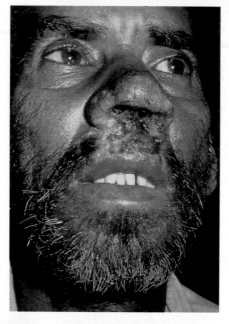

Figure 7.32 Paracoccidioidomycosis. Destructive lesion, philtrum and nose.

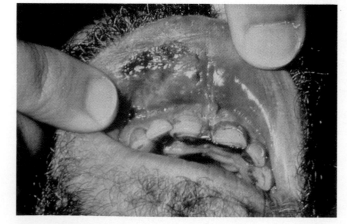

Figure 7.33 Paracoccidioidomycosis. Ulcerations, lip and buccal mucosa.

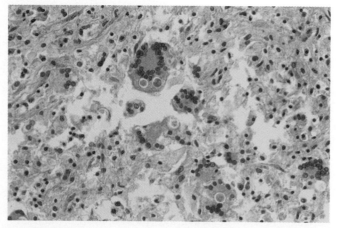

Figure 7.34 Paracoccidioidomycosis. Skin biopsy, hematoxylin-eosin stain. *Paracoccidioides brasiliensis*, mother cells within multinucleate giant cells. Buds are not evident.

medium are wooly, gray, green, yellow-green, or yellow-orange and produce a bright red pigment that diffuses into the medium (Figs. 7.35 and 7.36). Hyphae are hyaline, producing lateral, smooth-surfaced conidiophores that bear metulae, tapered phialides, and lemon-shaped conidia (Figs. 7.37 and 7.38).

At 37°C, colonies are white to tan and wrinkled, with less pigment production. Cells are yeast-like, are oval or elliptical, and divide by fission.[2,17]

Clinical Features

Penicilliosis (*P. marneffei*) is an opportunistic infection reported with increasing frequency in HIV-positive patients who reside in Southeast Asia or have visited the area. It is now considered an AIDS-defining event, although similar infections have been reported in patients with other forms of immunosuppression and even in individuals with no apparent immunodeficiency.

The disease mimics histoplasmosis. Individuals of all ages are susceptible. Portal of entry is probably pulmonary by aerosol inhalation. Signs and symptoms include fever, weight loss, cough, adenopathy, skin lesions, hepatosplenomegaly, and anemia. Bone, pericardial, and gastrointestinal involvement have also been observed.

Skin or mucosal lesions occur in 60 to 70% of patients. They are of great importance as convenient and rewarding sources of biopsy and culture material. Among the most common are papular lesions, sometimes few in number, nondescript, and easily over-

Figure 7.35 Penicilliosis (*Penicillium marneffei*). Culture at room temperature, Sabouraud's medium. Note the red pigment diffusing into the medium.

Figure 7.36 Penicilliosis (*Penicillium marneffei*). Culture at room temperature, Sabouraud's medium. Colony reverse.

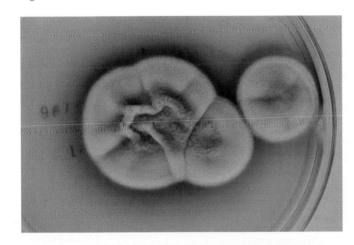

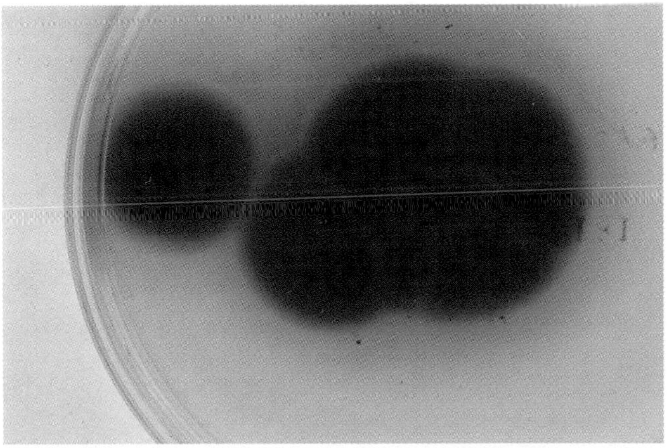

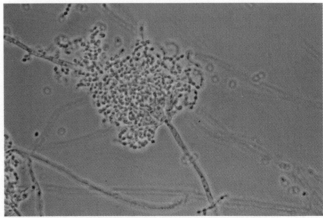

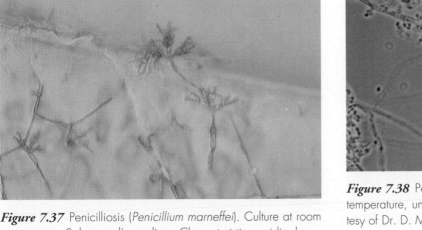

Figure 7.37 Penicilliosis (*Penicillium marneffei*). Culture at room temperature, Sabouraud's medium. Characteristic conidiophores and heads.

Figure 7.38 Penicilliosis (*Penicillium marneffei*). Culture at room temperature, undisturbed head. Lactophenol preparation. (Courtesy of Dr. D. McGinnis.)

looked. In other cases, they are multiple and widespread, often with delled or necrotic centers (Fig. 7.39). They may resemble molluscum contagiosum. Mucosal ulcers, cutaneous abscesses, pustular lesions, and nongenital cutaneous ulcers are also frequently observed. Genital ulcers, acneiform lesions, and lesions of the palate and oropharynx may occur and are usually seen in HIV-infected individuals.[17–20]

Pathology

As in histoplasmosis, a mixed dermal infiltrate is present in which neutrophils predominate. The yeast-like forms of the organism, round or oval and 3 to 4 μm in diameter, are packed into macrophages or lie free. Elongated sausage-shaped cells up to 8 μm in length, often with cross walls, also lie free. Budding does not occur. In tissues other than skin and lungs, reaction tends to be granulomatous. Focal necrosis and numerous extracellular yeast forms characterize the pattern often seen in immunocompromised individuals (Fig. 7.40).

Diagnosis

A history of travel to the endemic areas should alert the clinician. A presumptive diagnosis can be made with the demonstration of the characteristic nonbudding, cross-walled yeast forms in biopsy material. Definitive diagnosis depends on isolation of *P. marneffei* in culture. Blood, bone marrow, skin lesions, and sputum yield the highest percentages of positive results.

Treatment

Untreated penicilliosis (*P. marneffei*) is uniformly fatal. It is essential that antifungal treatment be administered promptly, especially in immunocompromised individuals. All consenting patients with penicilliosis should be tested for HIV infection.

Amphotericin B remains the medication of choice, alone or in combination with 5-fluorocytosine. (See the section on histoplasmosis for details on the administration of amphotericin B.) Therapy is continued for weeks or months. Relapse is common.

Ketoconazole and especially itraconazole are acceptable alternatives. The latter is administered in doses of 200 mg PO bid, with treatment to be monitored and continued for months. Relapse is common when the medication is discontinued. Indefinitely prolonged suppressive treatment with itraconazole is recommended for immunocompromised patients.[17–20]

The effectiveness and the optimum dosage and time schedules for treatment of this and other systemic mycoses with the newer antifungals have not yet been firmly established. Moreover, deleterious drug interactions have been observed with several of these medications. Clinicians are urged to consult the latest literature for guidance.

Differential Diagnosis

Miliary tuberculosis, lymphoma, and disseminated histoplasmosis, coccidioidomycosis, or cryptococcosis can be mimicked by penicilliosis (*P. marneffei*). Demonstration of the causative organism serves to establish the proper diagnosis.

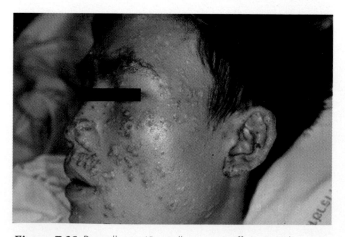

Figure 7.39 Penicilliosis (*Penicillium marneffei*). Papular eruption, face and ear. Note the central delling and necrosis. The patient is HIV-positive. (Courtesy of Dr. S. Chiewchanvit.)

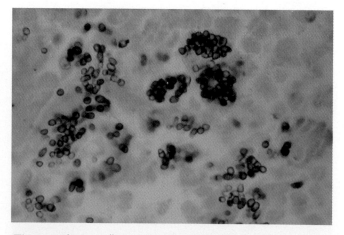

Figure 7.40 Penicilliosis (*Penicillium marneffei*) in the lung showing yeast-like forms that reproduce by fission. Gomori's methenamine silver stain. (Courtesy of Dr. S. Chiewchanvit.)

REFERENCES

1. Rippon JW; Histoplasmosis p 381 423. In: Medical Mycology. 3rd Ed. WB Saunders, Philadelphia, 1988

2. Crissey JT, Lang H, Parish LC: Disease caused by thermally dimorphic fungi. p. 115. In: Manual of Medical Mycology. Blackwell Scientific Publications, Cambridge, MA, 1995

3. Kwon-Chung KJ, Bennet JE: Histoplasmosis. p. 464. In: Medical Mycology. Lea & Febiger, Philadelphia, 1992

4. Wheat LJ: Histoplasmosis in Indianapolis. Clin Infect Dis 14, suppl. 1:S91, 1992

5. Wheat LJ: Endemic mycoses in AIDS: a clinical review. Clin Microbiol Rev 8:146, 1995

6. Kintzel PE, Smith GH: Practical guidelines for preparing and administering amphotericin B. Am J Hosp Pharm 49:1156, 1992

7. Wheat J, Hafner R, Korzun AH et al: Itraconazole treatment of disseminated histoplasmosis in patients with the acquired immunodeficiency syndrome: AIDS Clinical Trial Group. Am J Med 98:336, 1995

8. Galgiani JN: Coccidioidomycosis. West J Med 159:153, 1993

9. Jones JL, Fleming PL, Ciesielski CA et al: Coccidioidomycosis among person with AIDS in the United States. J Infect Dis 171:961, 1995

10. Galgiani JN, Catanzaro A, Cloud GA et al: Fluconazole therapy for coccidioidal meningitis. Ann Intern Med 119:28, 1993

11. Pappas PG, Threlkeld MG, Bedsole GD, Gelfand MS, Dismukes WE: Blastomycosis in immunocompromised patients. Medicine (Baltimore) 72:311, 1993

12. Witzig RS, Hoadley DJ, Greer DL, Abriola KP, Hernandez RL: Blastomycosis and human immunodeficiency virus: three new cases and review. South Medical J 87:715, 1994

13. Dismukes WE, Bradsher GC, Jr, Cloud CA et al: Itraconazole therapy for blastomycosis and histoplasmosis. Am J Med 93:489, 1992

14. Restrepo A: *Paracoccidioides brasiliensis.* p. 2028. In Mandell GL, Douglas RD, Bennett JE (eds): Principles and Practice of Infectious Diseases. 3rd Ed. Churchill Livingstone, New York, 1990

15. Negroni R: Paracoccidioidomycosis (South American blastomycosis, Lutz's mycosis). Int J Dermatol 32:847, 1993

16. Brummer E, Castenada E, Restrepo A. Paracoccidioidomycosis: an update. Clin Microbiol Rev 6:89, 1993

17. Wortman P: Infection with *Penicillium marneffei.* Int J Dermatol 35:393, 1996

18. Chiewchanvit S, Mahanupab P, Vanittanakon N: Cutaneous manifestations of disseminated *Penicillium marneffei* mycosis in five HIV-infected patients. Mycoses 34:245, 1991

19. Hilmarsdottir I, Meynard JL, Rogeaux O et al: Disseminated *Penicillium marneffei* infection associated with human immunodeficiency virus: a report of two cases and a review of 35 published cases. J Acquir Immune Defic Syndr 6:466, 1993

20. Sirisanthana V, Sirisanthana T: Disseminated *Penicillium marneffei* infection in human immunodeficiency virus–infected children. Pediatr Infect Dis J 14:925, 1995

CHAPTER 8

Staphylococcal Infections

Raza Aly

SUMMARY

Etiology Ten different species of *Staphylococcus* live on human skin (*S. aureus, S. epidermidis, S. hominis, S. haemolyticus, S. capitis, S. warneri, S. saprophyticus, S. cohenii, S. xylosus, S. simulans*); *S. aureus* is the most important etiologic agent

Clinical Features Impetigo, bullous impetigo, folliculitis, furuncles and carbunculosis, staphylococcal scalded skin syndrome

Diagnosis Clinical, histologic, and microbiologic methods

Treatment Antibiotic therapy

Differential Diagnosis Impetigo (other vesicular and pustular lesions); folliculitis (*Malassezia furfur* folliculitis, tinea barbae); furuncles and carbunculosis (herpes simplex, vaccinia, anthrax, tularemia, conglobate acne, hidradenitis); staphylococcal scalded skin syndrome (toxic epidermal necrolysis, viral infections, graft-versus-host infections)

Staphylococci are currently classified according to specific combinations of phenotypic characteristics and DNA relatedness. At least 10 different species of *Staphylococcus* live on human skin.[1] These include *S. aureus, S. epidermidis, S. hominis, S. haemolyticus, S. capitis, S. warneri, S. saprophyticus, S. cohenii, S. xylosus,* and *S. simulans.* The clinically most important is *S. aureus* (Table 8.1). Colonies of *S. aureus* on blood agar are surrounded by clear zones of hemolysis (Fig. 8.1). The microscopic appearance of gram-positive cocci arranged as large numbers of irregular clusters suggests staphylococci (Fig. 8.2).

The chief sites of *S. aureus* colonization are the anterior nares, perineum, axilla, and toe webs. Nasal carriage of *S. aureus* in nonhospital populations is generally about 10 to 45%.[2] Although *S. aureus* is rare on normal healthy skin, it is common on the skin of patients with dermatitis. Dermatitic skin, particularly atopic dermatitis, provides favorable ecologic conditions for *S. aureus* colonization.[3]

Folliculitis, furuncles, and carbuncles represent a continuum of severity of pustular lesions centered on a hair follicle (Fig. 8.3). The most common of all staphylococcal skin infections, folliculitis, is the result of infection of the hair follicle itself. When there is involvement of the subcutaneous tissue in addition to the follicle, the lesion is termed a furuncle or boil. In the neck and upper back, where the skin is thicker and less elastic, the infection may involve large areas, known as a carbuncle. In newborn infants, pustules or impetiginous lesions are the most frequent staphylococcal manifestations. These pustules may progress to extensive bullous impetigo. A severe form of staphylococcal infection of infants, the staphylococcal scalded skin syndrome, is induced by *S. aureus* belonging to group 2 phage types.

IMPETIGO

Impetigo is a contagious superficial infection of the skin initiated by *S. aureus* or group A β-hemolytic streptococci. Two diverse forms are recognized on the basis of bacteriologic, clinical, and histologic findings.[4,5] In superficial or common impetigo, the lesions are characterized by thick, adherent, and recurrent dirty yellow crusts with an erythematous margin. Superficial impetigo is the most familiar skin infection of children (see Ch. 9). Bullous impetigo is characterized by a superficial, thin-walled, bullous lesion that ruptures and develops a thin, transparent, varnish-like crust (Fig. 8.4).

Table 8.1 Staphylococcal Infections

MICROORGANISM	DISEASE
Staphylococcus aureus	Folliculitis, furuncle, carbuncle, bullous impetigo, staphylococcal scalded skin syndrome
Streptococcal pyogenes or *Staphylococcus aureus*	Superficial impetigo, blistering distal dactylitis

Figure 8.1 Colonies of *Staphylococcus aureus* on blood agar. Note clear zones of hemolysis around the colony.

Figure 8.2 *Staphylococcus aureus.* Gram stain from a 24-hour culture.

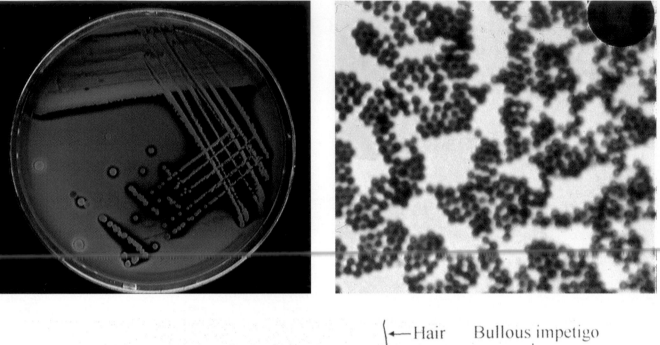

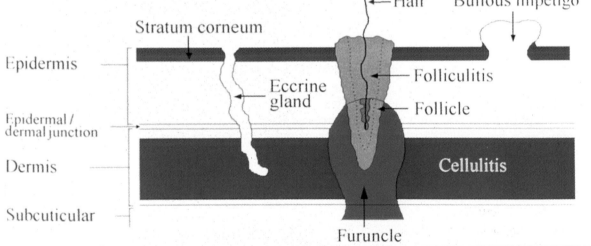

Figure 8.3 Continuum of pyodermas. *Staphylococcus aureus* folliculitis, furuncles, and carbuncles represent a continuum of severity of pustular lesions centered on a hair follicle. (Courtesy of Dr E. Epstein.)

BULLOUS (STAPHYLOCOCCAL) IMPETIGO

Etiology

The etiologic agent is *S. aureus*. The bullae are the result of local dyshesion of keratinocytes brought about by the action of the epidermolytic toxin (exfoliatin) elaborated by *S. aureus*.

Clinical Features

The frequency of this disease has been increasing since 1970. Its lesions are clinically characteristic.[4] Bullae are thin-walled, usually flaccid, but occasionally tense. They are easily ruptured and contain fluid ranging from a thin, cloudy, amber liquid to an opaque, white or yellow pus. After rupture of the bullae, the moist erythematous base dries quickly to form a thin, shiny, varnish-like veneer, which differs from the "stuck on" thicker crust of common impetigo. Lesions are most often found in groups in a single lesion (Fig. 8.5).

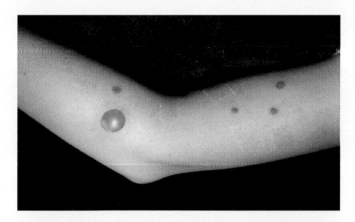

Figure 8.4 Bullous impetigo, a staphylococcal disease. (Courtesy of Dr. R. Odom.)

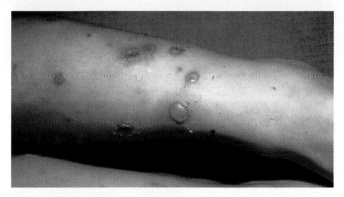

Figure 8.5 Bullous impetigo on the legs. Several lesions at different stages.

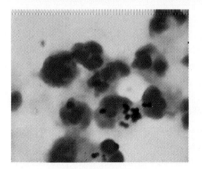

Figure 8.6 A Gram stain of a smear. Note the presence of gram-positive cocci.

Pathology

The presence of numerous neutrophils and the recognition of gram-positive cocci are characteristic of impetigo.

Diagnosis

The disease is diagnosed on the basis of characteristic bullae and is confirmed by Gram staining (Fig. 8.6) and culture.

Treatment

As in the case of impetigo, bullous impetigo should be treated with oral antistaphylococcal drugs (di-cloxacillin, a cephalosporin, or erythromycin) because these are more effective than topical antibiotic therapy. However, if the involvement is localized, topical antibiotics may be adequate. Indeed, the best topical agent, mupirocin, if applied three times daily for 7 to 8 days, is equivalent in efficacy to oral erythromycin. (see Chapter 9 for treatment of impetigo.) However, impetigo typically resolves even without treatment. The prognosis is excellent with immediate therapy. Septic complications are rare.

Differential Diagnosis

Bullous impetigo should be distinguished from other vesicular and pustular lesions.

**TREATMENT OF IMPETIGO
AND BULLOUS IMPETIGO**

Systemic Antibiotics
Erythromycin
Dicloxacillin
Cephalosporin

Topical Antibiotics
Mupirocin
Bacitracin
Neomycin-bacitracin combinations

FOLLICULITIS

Clinical Features

Folliculitis is infection of the epithelium of a hair follicle manifested by small erythematous follicular pustules without involvement of the surrounding skin. Most follicular infections involve multiple follicles (Fig. 8.7). The scalp and extremities are favored sites. Chronic recurrent folliculitis of the bearded area is termed sycosis barbae (barber's itch) (Fig. 8.8). Sycosis is usually propagated by the trauma of shaving and autoinoculation by the fingers.

The symptoms are slight burning, itching, and pain on manipulation of hair. The lesions are pustules centered on hair follicles. Consequently, each pustule may be pierced by a centrally located hair. In sycosis, the surrounding skin becomes involved, resembling eczema with redness and crusting.

Pathology

S. aureus growth in the ostium of the follicle may progress more deeply around the hair shaft with an accumulation of neutrophils.

Diagnosis

The typical lesions are manifested by small erythematous follicular pustules. The Gram stain of early lesions will show numerous cocci in clusters.

Treatment

The infected area should first be cleansed with a weak soap solution. This is followed by a daily soaking or compressing affected skin with saline or aluminium subacetate. When skin is softened, one can gently open the larger pustules and trim away necrotic tissue. Mixed ointment preparations containing polymyxin B, bacitracin, and neomycin can be effective when applied two to four times daily. Systemic antistaphylococcal antibiotics may be utilized if the skin infection is resistant; local treatment is in order if the scalp is involved. The disease can become stubborn, lasting for months or even years.

Differential Diagnosis

Folliculitis must be differentiated from M. furfur folliculitis and tinea barbae (Fig. 8.9) by microscopic examination of hair or by culture. Acne vulgaris and bullous impetigo may occasionally cause confusion. The patient's age and absence of comedones suggest a diagnosis of folliculitis instead of acne. The lesions of impetigo are usually larger.

FURUNCLES AND CARBUNCULOSIS

Etiology

A furuncle (boil) is an infection of the hair follicle with involvement of subcutaneous tissue (Fig. 8.10). Most are infected with S. aureus. The preferred sites of the furuncle are the hairy parts of skin exposed to friction and maceration. An inflammatory nodule develops topped by pustules through which a hair emerges. On the neck and upper back, multiple hair follicles may be involved, producing a carbuncle, which is defined as a large, indurated, painful nodule with multiple draining sites (Fig. 8.11). When infection occurs in the nasolabial area, extension via the vein draining into the cavernous sinus may lead to cavernous sinus thrombosis. Perinephric abscess, osteomyelitis, and similar hematogenous staphylococcal infection are other complications.

Clinical Features

Tenderness and pain are due to pressure on nerve endings, particularly in areas where there is little room for swelling of underlying tissues. Pain, fever, and malaise are more severe with a carbuncle than with a furuncle. The follicular abscess enlarges, becomes fluctuant, and then softens to open spontaneously, discharging a core of necrotic tissue and pus.

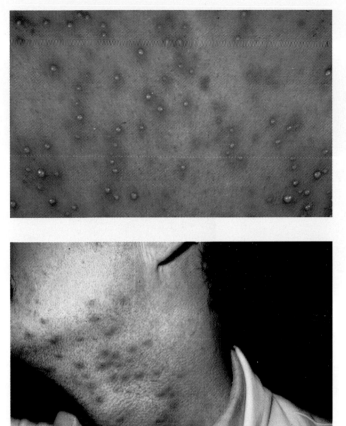

Figure 8.7 Folliculitis. The small papules are topped by superficial pustules located in the hair follicles.

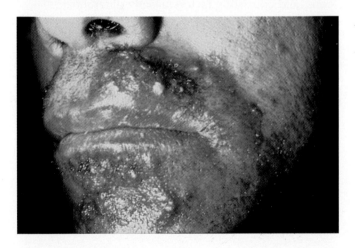

Figure 8.8 Sycosis barbae involving the bearded area.

Figure 8.9 Tinea barbae. The causative agent is a dermatophyte. Crusting and follicular pustules are similar to bacterial infections.

Diagnosis

Gram staining of pus will show gram-positive cocci in clusters.

Treatment

Local therapy Local care and sometimes surgical drainage of pus are sufficient to cure a majority of furuncles. The application of moist heat to developing abscesses or pustules hastens localization and aids in early and spontaneous drainage. A daily bath with antimicrobial soap is advisable. Clothing, including underwear, should be changed daily and thoroughly laundered.

Systemic Therapy Knowledge of antibiotic sensitivity of the organism is desirable for the selection of treatment.[3,6] About 80% of hospital strains of *S. aureus* in the United States are resistant to penicillin. Oxacillin, di-

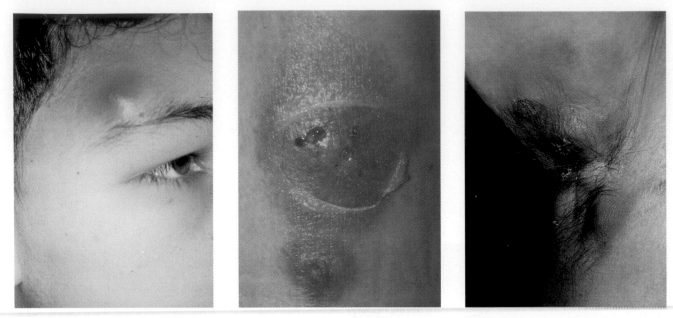

Figure 8.10 Furuncle. A single inflamed lesion near the eyebrow. The nodule is tender and painful.

Figure 8.11 Carbuncle. Two deeply seated lesions.

Figure 8.12 Hidradenitis suppurativa. Multiple abscesses in the axilla. Note one or more tender, abscess-like swellings in the apocrine gland area.

cloxacillin, nafcillin, and some cephalosporins are used in the treatment of these staphylococcal infections. Dicloxacillin (500 mg PO 6 h for 10 days) is generally effective.

Prevention

Control of recurrent furuncles can often be obtained by improving hygiene and by the elimination by systemic antibiotics. Some advocate treatment by bacterial interference. In this method, after effective antibiotic therapy, a relatively avirulent strain of *S. aureus* (502A) is deposited locally, preventing subsequent recolonization with a virulent strain. The procedure has been effective in controlling staphylococcal epidemics in newborn nurseries and in the management of patients with recurrent boils.[7] The practice of painting the nares of carriers with antibacterials, such as mupirocin, is also a helpful strategy in preventing recurrences.[8] In some patients, prognosis cannot be reliably determined during the first attack. Recurrent boils may affect the patient for months or years.

Differential Diagnosis

Differentiate from vesiculopustules of virus infections, such as herpes simplex and vaccinia, and from other bacterial infections, such as anthrax and tularemia. Conglobate acne and hidradenitis (Fig. 8.12) are infections of follicles, but their anatomic sites, multiplicity of lesions, and coexisting factors usually differentiate.

Prognosis

In some patients, prognosis cannot be reliably determined during the first attack. Recurrent boils may harass the patient for months or years.

STAPHYLOCOCCAL SCALDED SKIN SYNDROME

Etiology

Staphylococcal Scalded Skin Syndrome (SSSS) occurs mainly in infants and children. SSSS has also been called Ritter's disease or the malignant form of pemphigus neonatum.[9,10] Pathology ranges from localized bullae (as described in the section on bullous impetigo) to diffused exfoliative disease resulting from systemic toxemia. Epidermolytic toxin is produced by dermatopathic strains of *S. aureus*; it cleaves the epidermis longitudinally at the level of the stratum granulosum. Most often a purulent infection of the upper respiratory tract is present, but any purulent infection, like omphalitis, conjunctivitis, or impetigo, can play this role.

Epidermolytic toxin-producing strains belonging primarily but not exclusively to phage group 2 include types 55, 71, 3A, 3B and 3C. Investigators have shown that inoculation with living organisms results in impetigo, whereas injection of the isolated toxin induces localized scalding.

Clinical Features

The lesion is tender to the touch and has a rough, sandpaper-like texture. In the early phase, it is indistinguishable from the lesions of streptococcal scarlet fever, except for its tenderness. The lesions may first appear on the central portion of the face and the major body folds and then spread to the trunk and the extremities. In this erythematous stage, the Nikolski sign (i.e., seemingly normal skin wrinkles if gently rubbed) becomes positive. Within hours, spontaneous detachment of the skin

in large sheets takes place (Figs. 8.13 and 8.14). Bullae in this disease are so transient that diffuse erythroderma with large areas of exfoliation may be all that is seen. Bacterial toxemia, water loss, and electrolytic imbalance may result in hemodynamic shock and death. In some patients, the initial redness does not lead to peeling in large sheets, but, instead, is succeeded by a scaly desquamation.

Diagnosis

The skin splits intraepidermally, as demonstrated by microscopic examination of frozen sections of recently peeled skin. Cytologic smears of cells on the surface of denuded areas show cells of stratum granulosum (Tzanck smear). Cultures from intact bullae and other affected skin are generally sterile since the staphylococal infection can be found at the distant focal site. Nose, throat, conjunctiva or any impetigo area should be swabbed for bacterial culture.

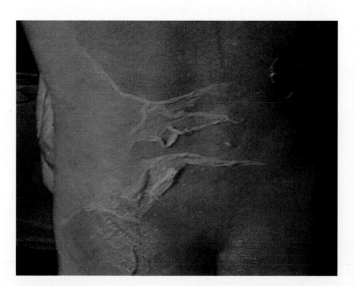

Figure 8.13 Staphylococcal scalded skin syndrome involving the whole body. Exfoliation occurs with separation of epidermis.

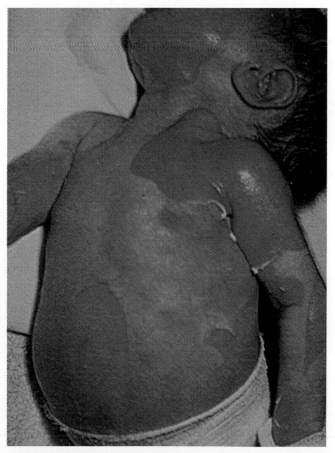

Figure 8.14 Staphylococcal scalded skin syndrome.

Differential Diagnosis

This disease can be confused with the idiopathic type of toxic epidermal necrolysis, which is associated with hypersensitivity reactions to drugs, with viral infections, and with the graft-versus-host reaction. In the idiopathic variety, the inflammatory response is intense, the epidermis is necrotic, and the cleavage plane develops either at the level of the dermal-epidermal junction or within the upper dermis. In SSSS, the skin separates in the granular cell layer.

Treatment

In severe cases, hospitalization of the patient is required. It is critical to be attentive to fluids and electrolyte balance. Treatment consists of administration of an oral penicillinase-resistant penicillin, such as dicloxacillin, 50 mg/kg/day in 4 divided dosages to a maximum of 2 g per day, or parenteral oxacillin or nafcillin at a dose of 75–100 mg/kg/day in divided doses intravenously every 6 hours, not to exceed 8 g per day. Corticosteroids should be avoided since they can delay resolution of the process.

Prognosis

The mortality is low provided that prompt therapy and proper measures are taken during the early phase of the disease. Although children with generalized SSSS typically recover, the syndrome in neonates and especially in adults is often fatal.

BLISTERING DISTAL DACTYLITIS

Blistering distal dactylitis is a distinctive infection usually associated with group A β-streptococci, although *S. aureus* is occasionally responsible (see Ch. 9). For staphylococcal lesions, dicloxacillin or erythromycin is recommended.[11]

REFERENCES

1. Kloos WE: Identification of *Staphylococcus aureus* and *Micrococcus* species isolated from human skin. p. 3. In Maibach HI, Aly R (eds): Skin Microbiology: Relevance to Skin Infection. Springer-Verlag, New York, 1981.

2. Williams RE: Healthy carriage of *Staphylococcus aureus*: its prevalence and importance. Bacteriol Rev 27:56, 1963

3. Aly R, Maibach HI, Shinefield HR: Microbial flora of atopic dermatitis. Arch Dermatol 113:780, 1977

4. Dillon HC: Impetigo contagiosa: suppurativa and non-suppurativa complications. Am J Dis Child 155:530, 1968

5. Darmstadt GL, Lane AT: Impetigo: an overview. Pediatr Dermatol 11:293, 1994

6. Demidovich CW, Wittler RR, Ruff ME et al: Impetigo: current etiology and comparison of penicillin, erythromycin and cephalexin therapies. Am J Dis Child 144:1313, 1990

7. Aly R, Shinefield HR, Maibach H: Bacterial interference among *Staphylococcus aureus* strains. p. 13. In Aly R, Shinefield HR (eds): Bacterial Interference. CRC Press, Boca Raton, FL 1982

8. Doebeling BN, Benenemen DL, Neu HC, et al: Elimination of *S. aureus* nasal carriage in health care workers: analysis of clinical trials with calcium mupirocin ointment. Clin Infect Dis 17:466, 1993

9. Lyell A: Toxic epidermal necrolysis: an eruption resembling scalding of the skin. Br J Dermatol 68:335, 1956

10. Elias PM, Fritsch P, Epstein EH: Staphylococcal scalded skin syndrome. Arch Dermatol 113:207, 1977

11. McCroy M, Esterley N: Blistering distal dactylitis. J Am Acad Dermatol 5:592, 1981

CHAPTER 9

Streptococcal Infections

Raza Aly

SUMMARY

Etiology Streptococcal skin infections are most commonly associated with group A streptococci

Clinical Features Superficial or common impetigo, scarlet fever, erysipelas, cellulitis, perianal streptococcal infection, blistering distal dactylitis

Diagnosis Clinical examination and culture techniques

Treatment Antibiotic therapies

Differential Diagnosis Impetigo (insect bites, herpes simplex, varicella-zoster, eczematous dermatitis, bullous disease); scarlet fever (rubella rubeola, drug eruptions, Kawasaki disease); erysipelas (cellulitis, erysipeloid); cellulitis (erysipelas); perianal streptococcal infection (psoriasis, seborrheic dermatitis, candidiasis, pinworm infestation, sexual abuse)

The nomenclature of streptococci, especially in medical use, has been based largely on serogroup identification of cell wall components rather than on species names. Skin infections are most commonly associated with group A streptococci (*Streptococcus pyogenes*). Streptococci are gram-positive cocci that occur in pairs or chains (Fig. 9.1). The ability to hemolyze erythrocytes aids in their classification; β-hemolytic streptococci produce complete lysis of the red blood cells surrounding the colony (Fig. 9.2). *S. pyogenes* is rarely seen on normal skin under hygienic conditions, although it may be carried in the throat of about 10% of the general population. The paucity of this microorganism on the skin is attributed to the presence of free skin lipids, which are lethal to streptococci. Cutaneous infections due to streptococci affect primarily the superficial layers of the epidermis but usually spare hair follicles. Deeper superficial streptococcal infections ulcerate down to the epidermal-dermal junction and scar after healing. Continuum of pyodermas due to *S. pyogenes* is illustrated in (Fig. 9.3).

SUPERFICIAL OR COMMON IMPETIGO

Common impetigo is more prevalent in hot, humid weather, which promotes the infection by providing greater opportunities for insect bites and other skin trauma on exposed extremities and by favoring bacterial growth on moist skin. Lack of personal hygiene and crowding are also predisposing factors.

Group A β-hemolytic streptococci and *Staphylococcus aureus* are found together or alone in common impetigo. Which organism is the primary pathogen remains controversial. One view is that common impetigo is streptococcal in origin with staphylococci as secondary invaders. Early lesions are more likely to yield pure cultures of streptococci; later lesions are apt to yield mixed cultures. As the lesion ages, staphylococci become more plentiful and easier to isolate. The other view is that common impetigo is initiated by either *S. aureus* or streptococci and that the *Staphylococcus*, being a more hardly organism, is encountered most frequently.

Clinical Features

Most lesions are found on exposed areas, particularly the face, scalp, and extremities (Figs. 9.4 to 9.6). The typical lesion begins as an erythematous papule in a

---

IMPORTANT PATHOGENIC STREPTOCOCCI

Group A streptococci
    Streptococcus pyogenes—beta hemolysis
Group B streptococci
    Streptococcus agalactiae—beta hemolysis
Group D streptococci
    Streptococcus bovis
    Enterococcus
Streptococcus pneumoniae
    Alpha hemolysis—has capsule, often occurs in pairs

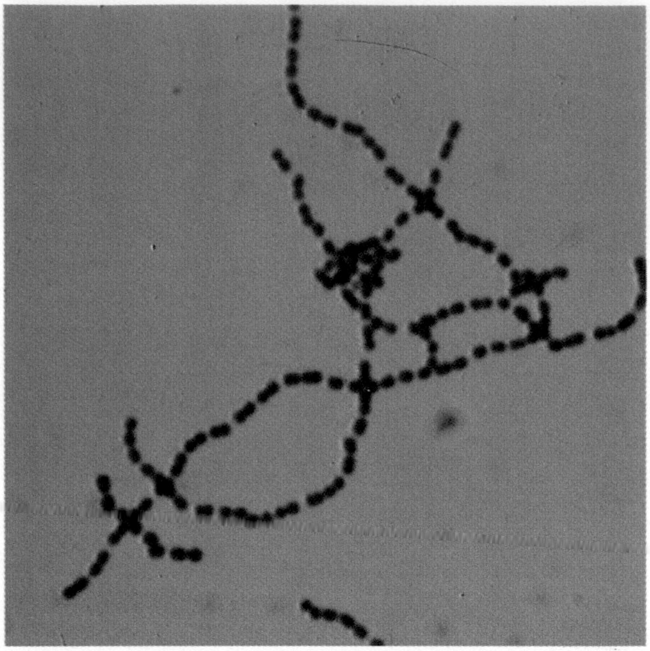

Figure 9.1 Group A streptococci. Note gram-positive cocci in chains.

Figure 9.2 Hemolytic streptococci. Note beta hemolysis around the colonies.

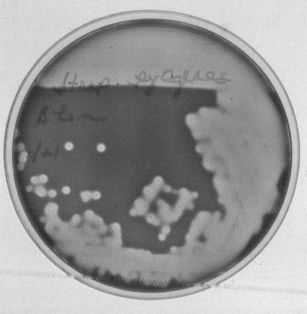

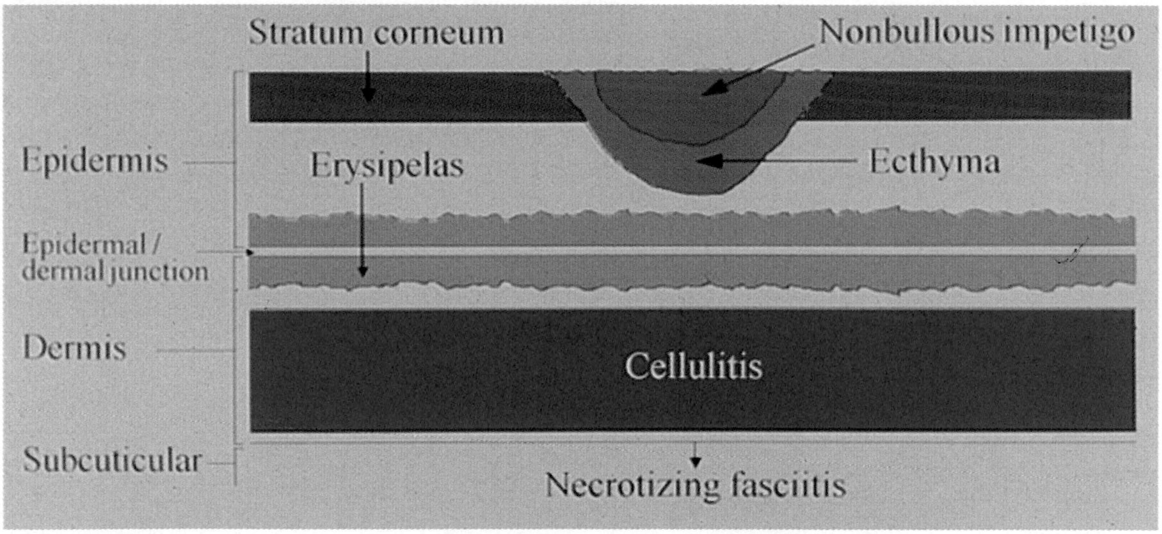

Stratum corneum

Nonbullous impetigo

Epidermis

Erysipelas

Ecthyma

Epidermal / dermal junction

Dermis

Cellulitis

Subcuticular

Necrotizing fasciitis

Figure 9.3 Continuum of pyoderma *Streptococcus pyogenes*.

traumatized area, such as an abrasion or insect bite. Small transient vesicles may develop, but the lesion rapidly evolves to its crusted form. The crust is adherent; upon its removal, a cloudy amber serous fluid exudes from the moist erythematous base. Punctuate, crusted, satellite lesions may surround the central lesion. Lesions may be discrete and limited initially, but with time they become multifocal and coalescent.

Diagnosis

The typical appearance of the thick, dirty-looking, honey-colored crust, along with itching, is almost pathognomonic of impetigo such that cultures generally are not needed before treatment is started. When the pus is aspirated from an intact pustule or vesicle, demonstration of organisms by Gram stain suggests a

Figure 9.4 Superficial impetigo in early stages, involving several localized areas.

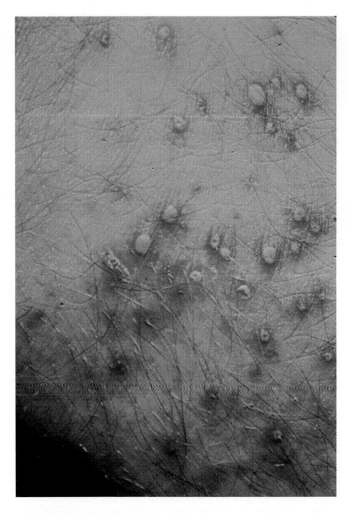

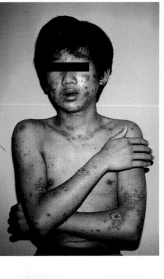

Figure 9.5 Superficial impetigo in later stages. Several crusts are formed. (Courtesy of Dr. R. Odom.)

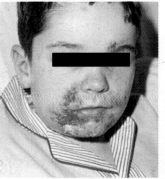

Figure 9.6 Superficial impetigo. Honey-colored crust is the hallmark of the disease.

pathogenic relationship (Fig. 9.7). Cultures and antibiotic sensitivity testing may be useful in evaluating patients who respond poorly to therapy.

Treatment

Treatment for impetigo should start with antistaphylococcal drugs because of coexisting *S. aureus* infections in many circumstances (Figs. 9.8 and 9.9). Oral dicloxacillin, cephalosporin, or erythromycin for 10 days has been demonstrated to be superior to local therapy. Dicoxacillin, 500 mg po q6h for 10 days in adults, is recommended. In children, 50 mg/kg/day, not to exceed 2 g/day, should be given in divided doses every 6 hours. When the patient cannot tolerate dicloxacillin because of penicillin allergy, erythromycin, 250 mg po q6h, can be substituted. Mupirocin (Bactroban) ointment is recom-

mended for the topical treatment of localized impetigo and pyodermas.[1] Clarithromycin, clindamycin, and cephalosporins such as cephalexin, cefacor, cefadroxil, or cefpodoxime are other choices.

Cleanliness and prompt attention to skin trauma can help prevent impetigo. Patients with impetigo and their families should be taught to bathe regularly with soaps containing antibacterial agents and to apply topical antibiotics to insect bites, cuts, abrasions, and infected lesions as soon as they are noted. Impetigo in infants is highly contagious and requires prompt treatment.

Differential Diagnosis

Many skin diseases that weep may suggest impetigo. These include insect bites, viral disease (herpes simplex, varicella-zoster), eczematous dermatitis, and bullous dis-

Figure 9.7 Demonstration of streptococci in a direct smear. Note cocci in chains.

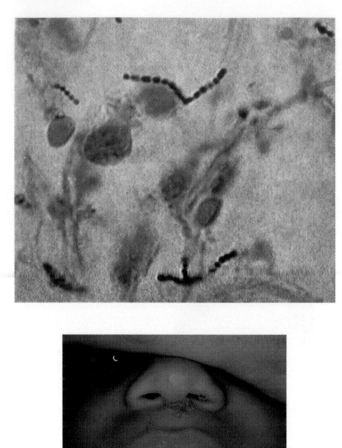

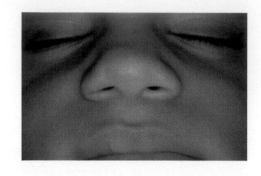

Figure 9.9 The same child seven days after treatment. The cultures were negative for group A streptococci and *S. aureus*. (Courtesy of Dr. P. Mertz.)

ECTHYMA

Ecthyma is a deeper form of impetigo. Lesions occur mainly on the legs and other covered areas often as a consequence of debility and infestation. Group A streptococci initiate the disease or complicate preexisting superficial ulcers.

The initial lesion is a vesicle or vesiculopustule with an erythematous base and surrounding halo, which enlarges and in a few days becomes thickly crusted. The ulcer has a "punched-out" appearance when crusts and purulent materials are removed (Fig. 9.10). The lesions are slow to heal, leaving scars.

Erythromycin or dicloxacillin given orally is effective (see section on impetigo for dosage schedule). Local treatment should consist of soaks and removal of crusts.

Figure 9.8 Impetigo. Exudative crusty lesions in a 5-year-old girl. Both *Staphylococcus aureus* and group A β-hemolytic streptococci were cultured. (Courtesy of Dr. P. Mertz.)

eases. *S. aureus* is frequently isolated as a secondary invader. The history, distribution, and morphologic features of primary lesions provide the best help for diagnosis of these other conditions. Lesions of herpes simplex are located to one anatomic site. Varicella has widely distributed lesions with uniform 2- to 3-mm vesicles.

Prognosis

Superficial impetigo generally has a good prognosis. Post-streptococcal glomerulonephritis rarely follows impetigo. Certain nephritogenic streptococci (types 49, 2, 55, 56, and 31) have been prevalent in impetigo resulting in nephritis. The anti-DNase B level is significantly elevated in patients with streptococcal impetigo, especially those with nephritis, but the ASO titer is usually normal.

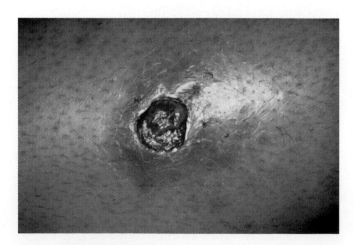

Figure 9.10 Ecthyma on the lower leg. The ulcer has a punched-out appearance.

SCARLET FEVER

Etiology

Scarlet fever results from strains of group A streptococci that produce erythrogenic toxin in patients who lack antitoxin immunity. The disease follows streptococcal pharyngitis or tonsillitis. In rare instances, it can be associated with skin and soft tissue infection. The disease is most prevalent in late fall, winter, and early spring.

Clinical Features

The onset of the disease is sudden and severe, starting after 2 to 4 days of incubation with headaches, fever, sore throat, and vomiting. Within 1 to 3 days later, the ex-anthem typically starts as an erythematous blush on the neck beneath the ear, on the chest, and in the axilla, quickly spreading to the abdomen, extremities, and face (Figs. 9.11 and 9.12). Petechiae are present in creases of elbows, groin, and axillary folds (Pastia's lines). The pharyngeal area, including the tonsils, is edematous, red, and beefy in appearance. The tongue is usually coated white with prominent bright red papillae, particularly on the lateral margin (strawberry tongue) (Fig. 9.13).

Diagnosis

A reliable diagnosis can be made on the basis of clinical findings and skin tests (Dick test and the Schulz-Charlton blanching test) and is confirmed by positive bacteriologic culture.

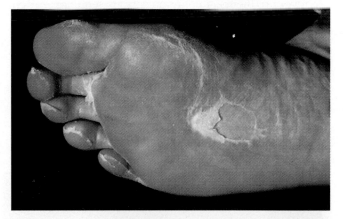

Figure 9.12 Scarlet fever. Involvement of the foot.

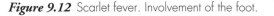

Figure 9.11 Scarlet fever. Exanthem of scarlet fever on the face.

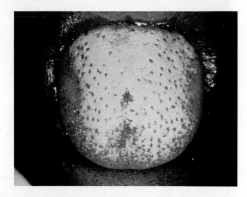

Figure 9.13 White strawberry tongue with prominent bright red papillae.

Treatment

Benzathine penicillin G and oral penicillin are preferred; erythromycin is the second choice. With benzathine penicillin G, adults are injected IM with 1.2 million U in a single dose; for older children, a single injection of 900,000 U is appropriate; and for infants and children weighing less than 27.3 kg, a single dose of 50,000 U/kg is usually sufficient.

Differential Diagnosis

The differential diagnosis includes viral infections (rubella, rubeola), drug eruptions (sulfonamides), and Kawasaki disease.

Prognosis

Because of the availability of effective antibiotic therapy, such complications as arthritis and jaundice are rare. Acute hemorrhagic glomerulonephritis and acute rheumatic fever are the most common serious sequelae.

ERYSIPELAS

Etiology

Erysipelas is an acute type of cellulitis of the skin and subcutaneous tissues.[2,3] This disease is contagious but does not produce explosive epidemics like those of scarlet fever. Erysipelas arises when group A β-hemolytic streptococci enter the skin. Sometimes other groups of streptococci (G and C) are associated.[4]

Clinical Features

For many clinicians, the term *erysipelas* applies solely to facial involvement. The disease is more common in the elderly. It may occur following facial injury or without any apparent cause and typically affects the cheeks, often spreading across the nasal bridge to form a butterfly pattern. Various clinical manifestations are shown in (Figs. 9.14 to 9.16).

Following an incubation period of 5 to 7 days, the abrupt onset of high fever is accompanied by headache, malaise, and vomiting. Lesions begin as small, bright red plaques that enlarge to about 10 to 15 cm in diameter. Erysipelas is characterized by raised,

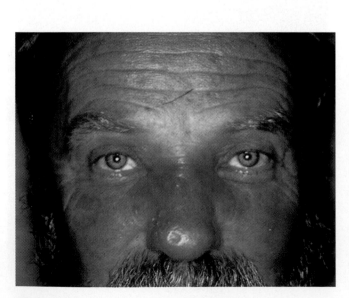

Figure 9.14 Erysipelas involving the face.

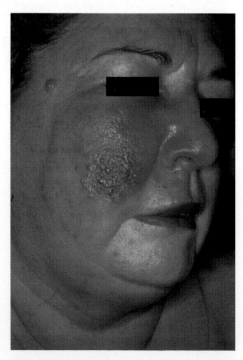

Figure 9.15 Erysipelas on the nose and cheek.

demarcated brilliant red areas. It may be painful or pruritic. Vesicles or bullae occasionally develop on the surface. Erysipelas is more superficial than cellulitis and predominantly affects the upper part of the dermis. Erythema and edema are sharply delineated in erysipelas, which contrast with the diffused edge of general cellulitis.

Pathology

Features of erysipelas include dermal edema and lymphatic dilation with diffuse neutrophil infiltration and limited localization around blood vessels.

Diagnosis

A definitive bacteriologic diagnosis of erysipelas (and cellulitis) is difficult to make. The paucity of bacteria in the tissues suggests that most of the inflammatory reaction may be an immune response to bacterial antigens or toxins rather than the effect of intact living bacteria.[5] The microorganism may be isolated from the blood or from the advancing margin of the lesions. Anti-DNaase B is helpful in identifying *S. pyogenes* infection.

Treatment

Penicillin is the drug of choice and should be given by mouth or parenterally, depending on the severity of infection and the ability of the patient to take oral medication (see Cellulitis below). Erythromycin is the alternative in the penicillin-allergic individual. Bed rest, keeping the head upright with several pillows, and taking aspirin for pain and fever are helpful.

Differential Diagnosis

Erysipelas should be differentiated from cellulitis and from erysipeloid, an infection common in fishery workers and meat handlers.

Prognosis

Before the advent of antibiotics, the disease was life-threatening, particularly for infants and the elderly. With prompt attention and treatment, it is now more readily controlled.

CELLULITIS

Etiology and Clinical Features

Cellulitis is a diffused inflammation of loose, particularly subcutaneous connective tissue.[5] Cellulitis affects the deep dermis and subcutaneous fat. It commonly involves the extremities, especially the calf (Figs. 9.17 and 9.18). Infection occurs generally through a breach in the skin surface, but it may frequently arise in normal skin also. β-Hemolytic streptococci are the typical isolated agents of cellulitis.[6] The skin is hot, red, and edematous. The edge of inflammation is irregular. As in erysipelas, vesicles, bullae, and exudation of fluid from the surface of the lesion may be noted.

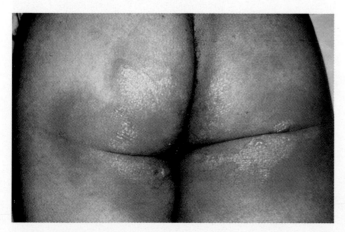

Figure 9.16 Erysipelas involving the buttocks and groin.

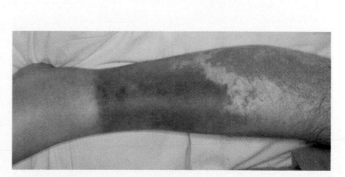

Figure 9.17 Cellulitis of the lower leg.

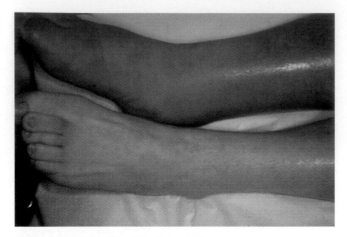

Figure 9.18 Cellulitis of the leg and foot.

Pathology

Features of cellulitis include dermal edema and lymphatic dilation with diffuse neutrophil infiltration and limited localization around blood vessels.

Treatment

Treatment is usually with penicillin, as discussed in the section on erysipelas. Although many clinicians believe that streptococci are the main microorganisms of cellulitis and therefore recommend penicillin, others are concerned about the possible role of *S. aureus*.

They instead advocate therapy active against both pathogens. Erythromycin and clindamycin are recommended when allergy to penicillin is suspected.[7] The affected inflamed area should be elevated to help reduce edema and support drainage of inflammatory products.

PERIANAL STREPTOCOCCAL INFECTION

Perianal streptococcal dermatitis is caused by the group A β-hemolytic streptococci.[8] There is perianal irritation, pruritus, tenderness, and painful defecation (Figs. 9.19 and 9.20). The differential diagnosis is psoriasis, seborrheic dermatitis, candidiasis, pinworm infestation, and sexual abuse. Oral penicillin in combination with topical mupirocin is recommended.[9]

BLISTERING DISTAL DACTYLITIS

Blistering distal dactylitis is a distinctive infection usually associated with group A β-hemolytic streptococci, although *S. aureus* is occasionally responsible. A tender, superficial bulla on an erythematous base develops on the volar fat pad of a finger or thumb and may extend to involve the hyponychial area (Fig. 9.21). The mi-

---

TREATMENT OF ERYSIPELAS AND CELLULITIS[A]

- *Bed rest and elevation of affected area.*
- *Application of cold compresses.*
- *Patients with complicated cellulitis should be hospitalized initially as parenteral therapy is needed.*

Use of Antibiotics
- *Intravenous penicillin for seriously ill patients*
  Alternates: cefazolin, clindamycin, vancomycin
- *Oral antibiotics for mild to moderate infections*
  Erythromycin
  Dicloxacillin
  Clindamycin
  Cephalexin

[a] Treat against both staphylococci and streptococci, unless Gram stain or cultures can be obtained.

(From Berger et al.,[7] with permission)

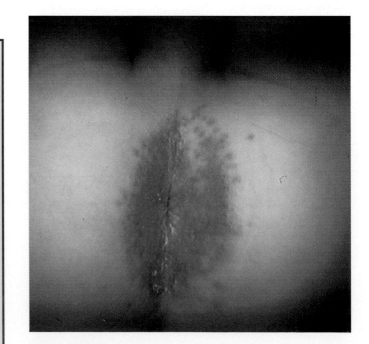

Figure 9.19 Perianal streptococcal infection.

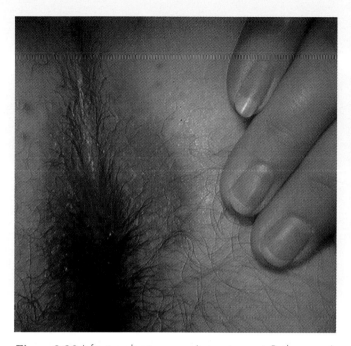

Figure 9.20 Infection due to group A streptococci. Both group A streptococci and *Staphylococcus aureus* were isolated. (Courtesy of Dr. D. Horney.)

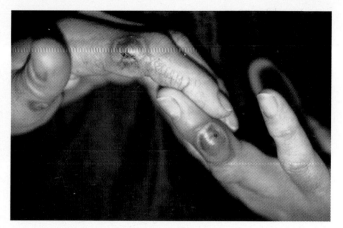

Figure 9.21 Blistering distal dactylitis. (Courtesy of Dr. T. Berger.)

croorganism is identified by gram-stained smears and culture of the blister fluid. Treatment consists of incision, drainage, compresses, and systemic penicillin. For staphylococcal lesions, dicloxacillin or erythromycin is recommended.[10]

REFERENCES

1. Britton JW, Fajardo JE, Krafte-Jacobs B: Comparison of mupirocin and erythromycin in the treatment of impetigo. J Pediatr 117:827, 1990

2. Maibach HI, Aly R: Bacterial infection of the skin. p. 710. In Moschella SL, Hurley JH (eds): Dermatology. 3rd Ed. WB Saunders, Philadelphia, 1992

3. Bernard P, Bedane C, Mounier M et al: Streptococcal cause of erysipelas and cellulitis in adults. Arch Dermatol 125:779, 1989

4. Chartier C, Grosshans E: Erysipelas. Int J Dermatol 29:459, 1990

5. Sachs MK: Cutaneous cellulitis. Arch Dermatol 127:493, 1991

6. Hook EW, Hooten TM, Horton CA et al: Microbiologic evaluation of cutaneous cellulitis in adults. Arch Intern Med 146:295, 1986

7. Berger T, Elias PM, Wintroub BU (eds): Manual of Therapy for Skin Diseases. Churchill Livingstone, New York, 1990

8. Amren DP, Anderson AS, Wannamaker LW: Perianal cellulitis associated with group A streptococci. Am J Dis Child 112:546, 1986

9. Krol LA: Perianal streptococcal dermatitis. Pediatr Dermatol 7:97, 1990

10. McCroy M, Esterly N: Blistering distal dactylitis. J Am Acad Dermatol 5:592, 1981

CHAPTER 10

Gram-Negative Infections: Folliculitis, Toe Web, Others

Guy F. Webster

SUMMARY

Etiology   Gram negative bacteria–*Pseudomonas*, *Escherichia*, *Klebsiella*, *Vibro* and *Proteus*.

Clinical Features   Vary from disease to disease.

Diagnosis   Clinical, direct microscopy and culture.

Treatment   Oral antibacterial agents, isotretinoin and topical medications (benzoyl peroxide and metronidazole).

Gram-negative bacteria are not typically stable members of the cutaneous microflora because of the relative dryness of the skin. There are individuals who harbor gram-negative bacteria on normal skin for a time, but true carriage in any area other than the toe webs, axilla, or groin is rare. For this reason, gram-negative infections in the absence of trauma or some unusual predisposing factor such as overhydration are uncommon.

The importance of hydration in skin ecology is illustrated by experiments in which normally dry forearm skin is occluded with plastic wrap. In a short time, the bacterial flora becomes more populous and assumes the character of the groin or axilla, with numerous gram-negative bacteria. Certain anatomic sites mimic this environment, such as the intertriginous areas as well as artificially hydrated locations such as the feet, and may have an overgrowth of gram-negative bacteria.[1-3]

PSEUDOMONAS INFECTIONS

Etiology and Clinical Features

The gram-negative bacteria most likely to exploit changes in the cutaneous microenvironment are members of the *Pseudomonas* genus. The most common infection from this group of bacteria is probably subungual, the so-called green nail syndrome. These infections are typically seen in individuals who have wet hands due to jobs as nurses, bartenders, or hairdressers. Typically the bacterial infection follows a dermatophyte or yeast infection, which creates an area of onycholysis that then remains continuously moist. The nail develops a green or yellow hue due to the pyocyanin pigment produced by the organisms. A paronychia may also develop.

The environment is frequently a source for *Pseudomonas* infections. Hot tub folliculitis is a *Pseudomonas aeruginosa* folliculitis acquired in contaminated hot tubs and whirlpools[4-6] (Figs. 10.1 and 10.2). Clinically there are a few to many pustules, often on the lower trunk, which are more often tender than pruritic. Lesions are a brighter red than typical staphylococcal folliculitis and have a larger zone of surrounding erythema. Gram stain of pus, which is often a bit viscous, reveals typical small, gram-negative rods and numerous neutrophils. Although usually self-limited, systemic spread has been reported.

Another source for *Pseudomonas* folliculitis are "loofah" sponges used by many for bathing and valued

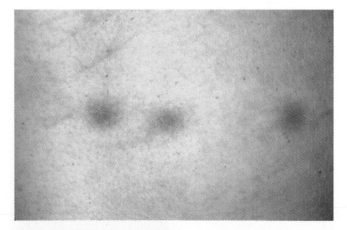

Figure 10.1 Cherry-red folliculocentric papules 2 days after bathing in a hot tub.

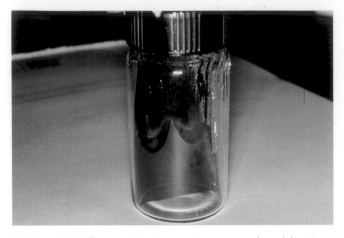

Figure 10.2 Characteristic green pigment produced by *Pseudomonas aeruginosa* in culture. In this case, "contaminating" growth on mycosal medium from a nail culture.

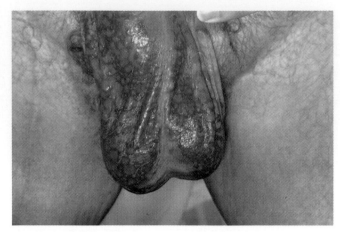

Figure 10.4 Chronic scrotal dermatitis overtreated with topical steroids and superinfected with *Pseudomonas.*

for the supposed benefit of exfoliating the skin[7,8] (Fig. 10.3). Actually dried gourds of the cucumber family, these sponges will harbor and actually serve as a growth substrate for *Pseudomonas,* which then is scrubbed into the skin. Infections with strains identical to those cultured from a patient's sponge have been documented. It is likely that other bathing aids that are not kept rigorously clean might also harbor gram-negative pathogens and serve as a means of infection (Fig. 10.4).

Treatment

Because the infection is fundamentally caused by an altered environment (moisture retained under onycholysis), specific antibacterial therapy is only temporarily useful unless the environment is restored to normal. Thus, antifungal therapy to cure any underlying infection is essential. Trimming away the distal separated

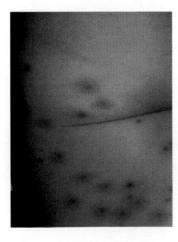

Figure 10.3 *Pseudomonas* folliculitis resulting from loofah sponge transmission.

portion of nail often provides sufficient drying to cure the *Pseudomonas* infection. Great benefit can also be derived from twice daily acetic acid soaks while the primary fungal infection is being treated with oral medications. Occasionally, in patients with severe diabetes or impaired circulation, it may be appropriate to treat the subungual *Pseudomonas* infection with oral antibiotics such as ciprofloxacin or trimethoprim-sulfamethoxazole to prevent a more severe infection.

MALIGNANT OTITIS

Malignant otitis is an otitis externa caused by *Pseudomonas* that has spread to cause a mastoiditis.[9–12] Patients are typically elderly, poorly controlled diabetics, and the disease may result in osteomyelitis, cranial nerve dysfunction, and even death. Besides pain and neurologic signs, the dermatologist may be alerted to the diagnosis by the presence of an exudative otitis externa, often confused with irritated seborrheic dermatitis. Diagnosis is made through a combination of physical examination, bacterial culture, and radiography of the mastoids. Intravenous therapy has been used traditionally, but newer fluoroquinolones may allow oral treatment in some cases.[13]

ECTHYMA GANGRENOSUM

Neutropenic patients may develop a macular eruption that quickly ulcerates and spreads circumferentially, which is a manifestation of *Pseudomonas* bacteremia. Patients are gravely ill, displaying classic signs of sepsis and disseminated intravascular infection including petechiae and purpura. Intravenous antibiotic therapy is mandatory, but even then mortality may approach 70%.

GRAM-NEGATIVE FOLLICULITIS IN ACNE

Etiology

Gram-negative superinfection of the face of acne patients was first recognized in 1968.[14] Patients typically have received long-term oral treatment for their acne with a tetracycline. Initially there is often a clear benefit to the acne therapy, but after months or years, pustules become unresponsive to the drug.

Clinical Features

Clinically the lesions are yellowish pustules with substantial surrounding erythema. Lesions are most common around the mouth and nose and may itch. When ruptured, the pus is quite viscous, and no comedo is detected. Various gram-negative organisms may be cultured including members of the genera *Klebsiella, Proteus, Pseudomonas, Escherichia, Serratia,* and *Citrobacter* (Fig. 10.5). *Proteus mirabilis* tends to cause deeper, more substantial lesions. Involved organisms can also be cultured from the nose, which may be the reservoir in this disease.[15]

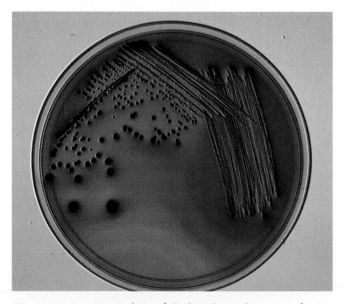

Figure 10.5 A pure culture of *Escherichia coli* growing from a gram-negative folliculitis pustule on MacConkey agar.

Treatment

The pathogenesis of gram-negative folliculitis involves the suppression of the cutaneous resident flora with antibiotic therapy, exposing the skin and nose to colonization by gram-negative organisms. Two therapeutic options exist: antibiotic or isotretinoin therapy. Patients may be treated empirically with trimethoprim-sulfamethoxazole or ciprofloxacin, usually with good results. More resistant disease responds well to isotretinoin in typical (0.5 to 1.0 mg/kg/day) dosages.[16]

VIBRIO VULNIFICUS INFECTIONS

A halophilic vibrio typically found in salt or brackish water, *Vibrio vulnificus* is increasingly recognized as an important human pathogen.[17] [19] The organism may infect wounds acquired in and around salt and brackish water and produces a rapidly spreading necrotizing cellulitis that may also display bullae. Occasionally no trauma is reported, but some marine exposure is the rule. Despite vigorous intervention including debridement and parenteral antibiotics, *V. vulnificus* infection may result in death, especially in some immunocompromised patients with diseases such as diabetes or liver disease. Diagnosis hinges on clinical suspicion and is confirmed later by positive cultures in appropriate salt-enriched media.

BACILLARY ANGIOMATOSIS

Etiology

In 1994, the first group of patients with bacillary angiomatosis were reported. All had acquired immunodeficiency syndrome (AIDS) and presented with superficial lesions resembling pyogenic granulomas or Kaposi's sarcoma.[20] There was a marked similarity to a rare tropical disease, Oroya fever, caused by *Bartonella bacilliformis.* Initial patients succumbed to infection and had widespread internal involvement, including one who had nodules occluding his airway.

The infection was soon found to be bacterial based on Warthin-Starry stains, but culture of the organism still proves difficult. Definitive bacterial identification currently relies on polymerase chain reaction identification of bacterial ribosomal RNA sequences in tissue.[21] The organism has had various names in the past few years, and taxonomists have finally settled on *Bartonella henslae.*[22,23]

Clinical Features

The vast majority of patients with bacillary angiomatosis are male patients infected with the human immunodeficiency virus (HIV) whose CD4 counts are less than 200/mm³. Occasionally an HIV-negative individual will manifest disease, but this is truly rare. Curiously, patients with Oroya fever are not known to be immunosuppressed, yet the two diseases are clinically similar and apparently caused by the same organism. Perhaps strain differences are involved. The geography of bacillary angiomatosis is also puzzling. Great variation in prevalence exists over relatively short distances. For example, it is common in lower Manhattan, less common in the northerly parts of that island, and almost nonexistent in Philadelphia. Adding to the confusion is the finding that the organism is carried by a high percentage of house cats,[24] but many patients have no cat exposure, and many AIDS patients with cats do not have the disease.

Cutaneous bacillary angiomatosis has three distinct lesion types, of which patients may display one or more.[25] The stereotypic lesion is a pinpoint red papule that grows to resemble a pyogenic granuloma or inflamed cherry angioma (Fig. 10.6). Lesions may be numerous or solitary and may be easily removed with a curette (without recurrence), leading to a great opportunity for misdiagnosis as angiomas. Deep-seated nodules are a second lesion type (Fig. 10.7). Usually few in number, these firm, often hyperpigmented lesions are most often seen on the extremities. The center of these lesions may be necrotic, and multiple biopsies are often required to obtain diagnostic pathology. The third cutaneous form of bacillary angiomatosis resembles Kaposi's sarcoma and is a firm purplish plaque typically on the lower leg. It may coexist with Kaposi's lesions in the same patient, and not uncommonly the infection is discovered after a supposed Kaposi's sarcoma lesion fails to respond to therapy. Multiple biopsies are often required.

Systemic involvement with the infection is common. Patients may feel terrible, with fevers, sweats, anorexia, and weight loss; care must be taken not to dismiss these symptoms as a nonspecific result of AIDS. The liver and spleen may swell, and transaminases may rise. The pleura and myocardium may be infected, as may the parenchyma of these organs. Painful osteolytic lesions are not uncommon. Even the brain may be involved in rare instances.[23,26–30]

Treatment

Empiric trials initially revealed that the infection is extremely sensitive to the tetracyclines and macrolides. Oral therapy is usually sufficient. Cell wall active antibiotics, rifampin, sulfonamides, and fluoroquinolones are inactive or unreliable for therapy.[20,23]

ULCER INFECTIONS

Clinical Features

Chronic vascular ulcers or even chronically inflamed broken skin (e.g., stasis dermatitis or intertrigo) (Figs. 10.8 and 10.9) can become significantly colonized by gram-negative organisms, leading to local or distant infection.[31,32] The presence of moisture changes the cutaneous ecology enough to allow gram-negative proliferation. In these situations, it may be difficult to determine

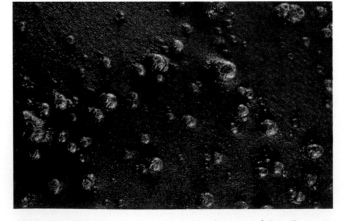

Figure 10.6 Pyogenic granuloma-like lesions of bacillary angiomatosis.

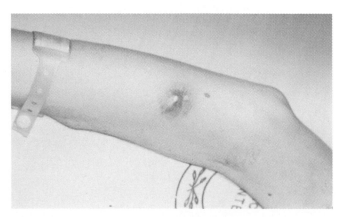

Figure 10.7 Nodular lesion of bacillary angiomatosis.

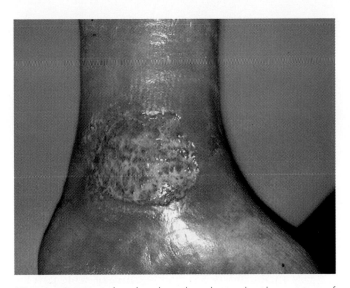

Figure 10.8 Vascular ulcer heavily colonized with a mixture of gram-negative organisms including *Escherichia coli*, *Pseudomonas aeruginosa*, and *Proteus mirabilis*. Surrounding erythema is sometimes an indicator of significant colonization.

at what point colonization becomes infection, since the clinical signs of infection (warmth, redness, swelling, pain) are already present due to the underlying inflammatory disease or wound. Significant colonization/infection can sometimes be detected by an increase in the severity of inflammation, for example, increased exudation of an ulcer. Another clue is foul odor. Gram-negative aerobes produce fruity (*Escherichia*, *Klebsiella*, *Pseudomonas*) or ammoniacal (*Proteus*) smells. Anaerobes such as *Bacteroides* produce fatty acid odorants with a more fecal note.

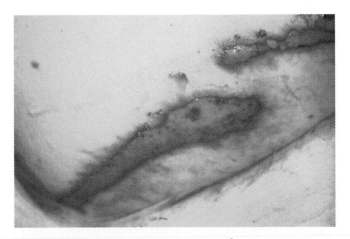

Figure 10.9 Ulcerated intertrigo in an obese patient that is secondarily infected with various gram-negative enteric bacteria.

Treatment

Therapy of gram-negative colonization of wounds is ultimately best accomplished by healing the wound. When this cannot be done quickly, the next best option is to alter the environment so that it is no longer supportive to colonization; that is, dry it out. In stasis dermatitis and venous ulceration, compressive treatments with bandages or pneumatic devices may be sufficient. Occasionally, antibacterial therapy is needed. Topical medications (e.g., benzoyl peroxide or metronidazole) are strongly preferred, since long-term treatment is usually needed and systemic therapy may ultimately result in generation of resistant gram-negative organisms in the ulcer.

REFERENCES

1. Noble WC: Infection with gram negative bacilli. Semin Dermatol 1:111, 1982

2. Marples RR: The effect of hydration on the bacterial flora of the human skin. p. 33. In Maibach HI, Hildick-Smith G (eds): Skin Bacteria and Their Role in Infection. McGraw-Hill, New York, 1965

3. Leyden JJ, McGinley KJ, Webster GF: Cutaneous microbiology. p. 1153. In Goldsmith L (ed): The Biochemistry and Physiology of the Skin. Oxford University Press, London, 1983

4. Ratnam S, Hogan K, March SB, Hutchison RH, Schaffner W: *Pseudomonas* folliculitis and outbreak and review. J Clin Microbiol 23:655, 1986

5. Price D, Ahearn DG: Incidence and persistence of *Pseudomonas aeruginosa* on whirlpools. J Clin Microbiol 26:1650, 1988

6. Thomas P, Moore M, Bell E et al: *Pseudomonas* dermatitis associated with a swimming pool. JAMA 253:1156, 1985

7. Bottone EJ, Perez AA: *Pseudomonas aeruginosa* folliculitis acquired through use of a contaminated loofa sponge: an unrecognized potential public health problem. J Clin Microbiol 31:480, 1993

8. Bottone EJ, Perez AA, Oeser JL: Loofa sponges as reservoirs and vehicles in the transmission of potentially pathogenic bacterial species to human skin. J Clin Microbiol 32:469, 1994

9. Chandler JR: Malignant external otitis. Laryngoscope 78:1257, 1968

10. Zaky DA, Bentley DW, Lowy K, Betts RF, Douglas RG: Malignant external otitis, a severe form of otitis in diabetic patients. Am J Med 61:298, 1976

11. Doroghazi RM, Nadol JB, Hyslop NE, Baker AS, Axelrod L: Invasive external otitis: a report of 21 cases and review of the literature. Am J Med 71:603, 1981

12. Johnson MP, Ramphal R: Malignant external otitis: report on therapy with ceftazidime and review of therapy and prognosis. Rev Infect Dis 12:173, 1990

13. Lang R, Goshen S, Kitzes-Cohen R, Sade J: Successful treatment of malignant external otitis with oral ciprofloxacin: report of experience with 23 patients. J Infect Dis 161:537, 1990

14. Fulton JE, McGinley KJ, Leyden JJ, Marples RR: Gram negative foliculitis in acne vulgaris. Arch Dermatol 98:349, 1968

15. Blankenship ML: Gram negative folliculitis, follow-up observations in 20 patients. Arch Dermatol 120:1301, 1984

16. Plewig G, Nikolowski J, Wolff HH: Action of isotretinoin in acne rosacea and gram negative folliculitis. J Am Acad Dermatol 6:766, 1982

17. Hill MK, Sanders CV: Localized and systemic infections due to *Vibrio* species. Infect Dis Clin North Am 1:687, 1987

18. Howard RJ, Bennett NT: Infections caused by halophilic marine vibrio. Ann Surg 217:525, 1993

19. Penman AD, Lanier DC, Avara WT et al: *Vibrio vulnificus* wound infections from Mississippi Gulf coastal waters: June to August 1993. South Med J 88:531, 1995

20. Cockerell CJ, Webster GF, Whitlow MA, Friedman-Kein AE: Epitheloid angiomatosis: a distinct vascular disorder in patients with the acquired immunodeficiency syndrome or AIDS-related complex. Lancet 2:654, 1987

21. Relman DA, Loutit JS, Schmidt TM et al: The agent of bacillary angiomatosis, an approach to the identification of uncultured pathogens. N Engl J Med 323:1573, 1990

22. Relman DA, Lepp PW, Sadler KN et al: Phylogenetic relationships among the agents of bacillary angiomatosis, *Bartonella bacilliformis*, and other alphaproteobacteria. Mol Microbiol 6:1801, 1992

23. Cockerell CJ: Bacillary angiomatosis and related diseases caused by *Rochalimaea*. J Am Acad Dermatol 32:783, 1995

24. Groves MG, Harrington KS: *Rochalimaea henslae* infections: newly recognized zoonoses transmitted by domestic cats. J Am Vet Med Assoc 204:267, 1994

25. Webster GF, Cockerell CJ, Friedman-Kien AE: The clinical spectrum of bacillary angiomatosis. Br J Dermatol 126:535, 1992

26. Baker J, Ruiz-Rodriguez R, Whitfield M et al: Bacillary angiomatosis, a treatable cause of acute psychiatric symptoms in HIV infection. J Clin Psychiatry 56:161, 1995

27. Moore EH, Russell LA, Klein JS et al: Bacillary angiomatosis in patients with AIDS: multiorgan imaging findings. Radiology 197:67, 1995

28. Conrad SE, Jacobs D, Gee J, et al: Pseudoneoplastic infection of bone in AIDS. J Bone Joint Surg [Am] 73:774, 1991

29. Garcia-Tsao G, Panzini L, Yoselevitz M et al: Bacillary peliosis hepatitis as cause of acute anemia in a patient with AIDS. Gastroenterology 102:1065, 1992

30. Slater LN, Min KW: Polypoid endobronchial lesions: a manifestation of bacillary angiomatosis. Chest 102:972, 1992

31. Galpin JE, Chow AW, Bayer AS, Guze LB: Sepsis associated with decubitus ulcers. Am J Med 61:346, 1976

32. Parish LC, Witkowski JA: The infected decubitus ulcer. Int J Dermatol 28:643, 1989

CHAPTER 11

Mycobacterial Infections

Lee T. Nesbitt, Jr.
Donald L. Greer

SUMMARY

Etiology Species of the genus *Mycobacterium* produce tuberculosis, nontuberculous infections, and leprosy.

Clinical Features Tuberculosis, nontuberculous mycobacterial infections. Clinical manifestations vary according to the immunologic status of the host.

Pathology Tuberculosis (tubercule), nontuberculous mycobacteria (variable pathology).

Diagnosis Histopathology and culture, polymerase chain reaction analysis (*Mycobacterium tuberculosis*).

Treatment Multidisciplinary approach and antituberculous regimen, surgical treatment (nontuberculous mycobacteria).

Species of the genus *Mycobacterium* produce most tuberculosis, nontuberculous mycobacterial infections, and leprosy. This chapter discusses cutaneous tuberculosis and infections caused by the nontuberculous (atypical) mycobacteria.

ETIOLOGY

Mycobacteria are acid-fast, weakly gram-positive rods. The modified Runyon classification of mycobacteria is presented in Table 11.1 and divides mycobacteria into slow-growing and rapidly growing organisms.

Infections due to *Mycobacterium tuberculosis* are classified according to the inoculation route, as shown in Table 11.2. The inoculation can occur from an exogenous source, from an endogenous source, or from hematogenous spread. Both the general immunologic state of the host and the specific host immunity to *M. tuberculosis* are factors in the type of skin lesions that will develop from each type of inoculation.

Nontuberculous mycobacteria, unlike *M. tuberculosis*, are not usually transmitted from person to person. These opportunistic organisms are found in many types of water and soil, with entry most often from direct inoculation. Less commonly, infection occurs by inhalation or ingestion. What causes these organisms to become pathogenic is not known, although immunosuppression of the host undoubtedly plays a role in the ability of many of these organisms to produce infection. However, the majority of infections caused by *Mycobacterium marinum*, the most common atypical mycobacterium that produces cutaneous disease, occur in immunocompetent persons.

Primary infections due to *M. tuberculosis* and nontuberculous mycobacteria may occur in immunocompetent individuals, usually with resolution of the infection, but immunosuppression facilitates spread or dissemination of the disease and may be what allows many nontuberculous organisms to become pathogenic.

CLINICAL FEATURES

Tuberculosis

Cutaneous tuberculosis is classified in Table 11.2. In the case of no prior exposure, a papulonodule will develop at the inoculated site with rapid evolution into a painless ulcer (tuberculous chancre). This is associated with prominent regional lymphadenopathy, similar to any chancriform complex. In most instances, the primary ulceration heals, followed by healing of the lymphadenopathy over many months.

If an inoculation occurs in a patient who has been previously exposed (post-primary inoculation) to *M. tuberculosis*, verrucous papules may develop at the site of exposure, sometimes with peripheral extension, which results in hyperkeratotic plaques (tuberculosis verrucosa cutis, warty tuberculosis). These lesions may extend slowly without treatment, may remain stable, or may heal spontaneously. Regional lymphadenopathy is not a feature of post-primary inoculation infection.

Cutaneous tuberculosis with contiguous spread (scrofuloderma) results from tuberculosis in deep tissues extending to the skin (Fig. 11.1). Most commonly, the extension is from lymph nodes, although bone, joint, or other organ tuberculosis may be the site of origin. The

Table 11.1 Classification of Pathogenic Mycobacteria

MYCOBACTERIUM SPECIES	RUNYON GROUP
Slow-growing mycobacteria	
Obligate human pathogens	
M. tuberculosis var. bovis group including bacillus Calmette-Guérin (BCG)	
M. africanum	
Facultative human pathogens	
M. kansasii	I
M. marinum	I
M. scrofulaceum	II
M. szulgai	II
M. avium-intracellulare complex	III
M. haemophilum	III
M. ulcerans	III
M. xenopi	III
Rapidly growing mycobacteria	
Facultative human pathogens	
M. fortuitum complex (M. fortuitum and M. chelonei)	IV

Note: *M. leprae* is not included in this table because it has not been grown in culture.

lateral aspects of the neck are the sites most often involved. Nodular skin lesions develop with breakdown of overlying skin and drainage of purulent or caseous material. Sinus tracts and ulcers develop with keloidal scarring as a common end result.

Autoinoculation tuberculosis (orificial tuberculosis) occurs on or around mucous membranes due to autoinoculation of *M. tuberculosis* from progressive disease in internal organs (Fig. 11.2). The mouth and perioral area are the most common sites involved, related to inoculation of organisms from the lower respiratory tract. Anal lesions may occur from intestinal tuberculosis and urethral or vulvar disease from proximal genitourinary involvement. Usually, a small nodule will appear that breaks down to form an irregular, punched-out ulcer with undermined edges. Lesions are extremely painful and may be single or multiple.

The most common form of cutaneous tuberculosis is lupus vulgaris, which is presumed to be related to silent hematogenous spread (Figs. 11.3 and 11.4). Organisms probably disseminate during the course of primary pulmonary infection with scattered inactive tuberculomas as a result. Lupus vulgaris lesions later develop from activated tuberculomas, and the process becomes an extremely chronic, progressive cutaneous disorder. The head and neck are involved in about 90% of cases, with the earlobes, nose, and cheeks commonly affected. Lesions usually begin as reddish-brown papules that evolve into plaques. When blood is pressed out of a lesion with a glass slide (diascopy), the characteristic apple-jelly color of lupus vulgaris is often evident. Scarring is a prominent feature of the disease, and in long-standing lesions, squamous cell carcinoma can occur.

Other rare forms of hematogenous dissemination include acute cutaneous lesions of miliary tuberculosis, seen in infants and young children who have lowered immunity, (Fig. 11.5), and tuberculous abscesses, which may form in immunosuppressed patients at sites of previous trauma (Fig. 11.6). With miliary tuberculosis, lesions usually appear as small erythematous macules or papules, which may be purpuric. They may develop a central area of necrosis with crusting. In general, these acute lesions of hematogenous dissemination indicate a poorer prognosis.

Nontuberculous Mycobacteria

Nontuberculous mycobacterial organisms most commonly produce inoculation skin lesions, pulmonary infections in older adults, cervical lymphadenitis in children, and disseminated disease in immunosuppressed individuals. Infections of the skin, soft tissues, lung, lymph nodes, bone, joints, eye, heart, and other organs have been reported. The spectrum of disease associated with nontuberculous mycobacteria is listed in Table 11.3.

M. marinum produces cutaneous disease more commonly than any other nontuberculous mycobacterium. This organism occurs in both saltwater and freshwater, including swimming pools and aquariums. Infection occurs after trauma to skin that is in contact with infected water from any of these sources. The color of the lesion is usually erythematous to violaceous, and some scaling is often present. The most common site of involvement is the skin over joints of the hands, feet, elbows, or knees (Figs. 11.7 to 11.11). Occasionally, a lymphangitic, sporotrichoid pattern of nodules develops along the lymphatic drainage of an extremity. These may suppurate and drain. Regional lymph nodes may also become enlarged but do not suppurate. Occasionally, penetration of the organism to an underlying bursa or joint may occur (Figs. 11.12 and 11.13), producing extracutaneous

Text continued on page 144

Figure 11.1 Contiguous spread tuberculosis (scrofuloderma). Draining sinuses from infected lymph nodes of the neck with keloidal-like scarring. (Courtesy of Dr. Lee T. Nesbitt, Jr.)

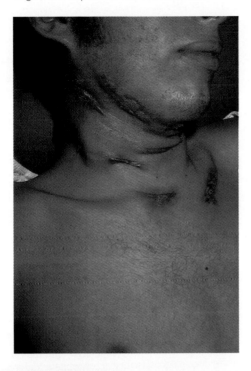

Figure 11.2 Autoinoculation (orificial) tuberculosis. Irregular ulcerative and eroded lesions of the perianal area secondary to gastrointestinal tract tuberculosis. (Courtesy of Dr. Lee T. Nesbitt, Jr.)

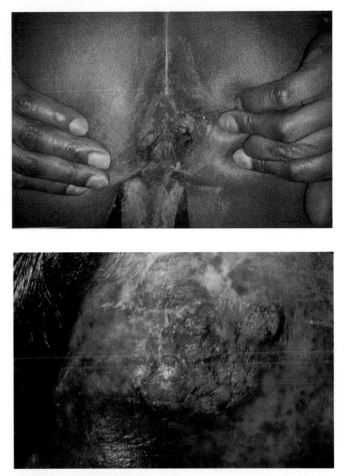

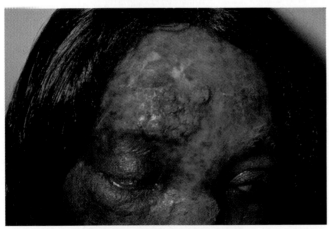

Figure 11.4 Lupus vulgaris. Close-up of lesion in Figure 11.3 showing ulcerative plaque with development of hyperkeratotic squamous cell carcinoma at right upper edge of lesion. (Courtesy of Dr. Lee T. Nesbitt, Jr.)

Figure 11.3 Lupus vulgaris. Chronic atrophic scarring of the forehead with active ulcerative plaque. (Courtesy of Dr. Lee T. Nesbitt, Jr.)

Table 11.2 Classification of Cutaneous Tuberculosis

CLASSIFICATION	SYNONYMS
A. Cutaneous tuberculosis from an exogenous source	
1. Primary inoculation	Tuberculous chancre Tuberculosis primary complex
2. Post–primary inoculation	Tuberculosis verrucosa cutis Warty tuberculosis Verruca necrogenica Prosector's wart
B. Cutaneous tuberculosis from an endogenous source	
1. Contiguous spread	Scrofuloderma Tuberculosis colliquativa cutis
2. Autoinoculation	Orificial tuberculosis Tuberculosis cutis orificialis Tuberculosis ulcerosa cutis et mucosae
C. Cutaneous tuberculosis from hematogenous spread	
1. Lupus vulgaris	Tuberculosis luposa cutis
2. Acute hematogenous dissemination	Acute miliary tuberculosis of the skin Tuberculosis cutis miliaris disseminata Tuberculosis cutis acuta generalista
3. Nodules or abscesses	Metastatic tuberculous abscess Tuberculous gumma

(Adapted from Beyt et al.: Cutaneous mycobacteriosis: analysis of 34 cases with a new classification of the disease. Medicine (Baltimore) 60:95, 1981)

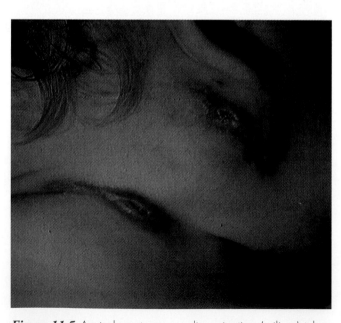

Figure 11.5 Acute hematogenous dissemination (miliary) tuberculosis. Erythematous ulcerative plaques of neck and posterior to ear in a child with acute disseminated tuberculosis. (Courtesy of Dr. Donald L. Greer.)

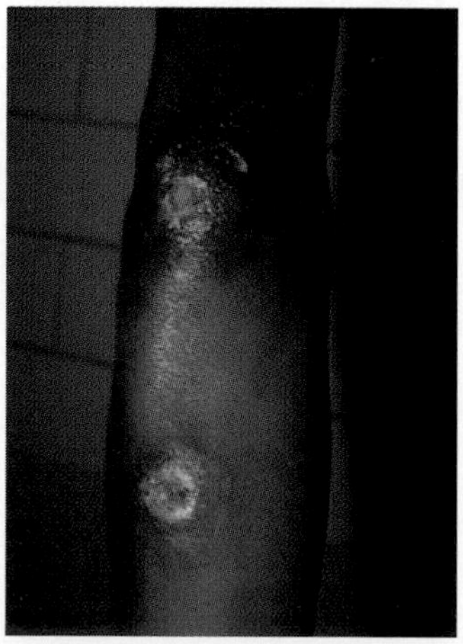

Figure 11.6 Tuberculous abscesses. Ulcerative nodules on back of arm in areas of trauma in patient with active systemic tuberculosis. (Courtesy of Dr. Lee T. Nesbitt, Jr.)

Figure 11.8 *Mycobacterium marinum* infection. Erythematous nodular plaques with multiple areas of inoculation on elbow. (Courtesy of Dr. Lee T. Nesbitt, Jr.)

Figure 11.7 *Mycobacterium marinum* infection. Erythematous, slightly ulcerated plaque on elbow of a child. (Courtesy of Dr. Lee T. Nesbitt, Jr.)

Figure 11.9 *Mycobacterium marinum* infection. Multiple erythematous to violaceous plaques on knee. Lesions simulate psoriasis.

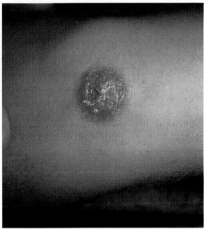

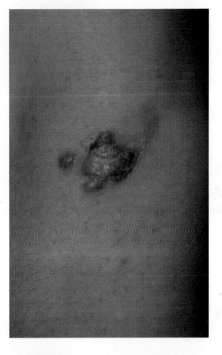

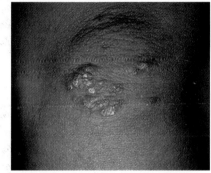

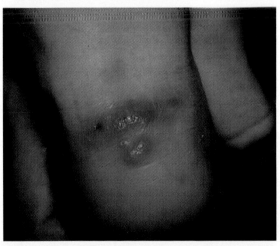

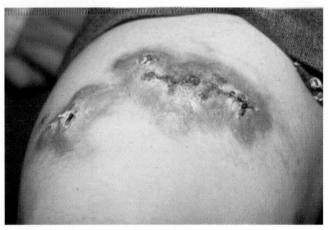

Figure 11.10 *Mycobacterium marinum* infection. Erythematous linear plaques on heel of a child from traumatic injury while swimming. (Courtesy of Dr. Lee T. Nesbitt, Jr.)

Figure 11.11 *Mycobacterium marinum* infection. Large violaceous and ulcerative plaques on leg from linear injury while in brackish waters. (Courtesy of Dr. Lee T. Nesbitt, Jr.)

Table 11.3 Nontuberculous Mycobacteria: Usual Spectrum of Disease

DISEASE	MOST COMMON MYCOBACTERIUM SPECIES
Chronic pulmonary infection	M. avium-intracellulare complex
	M. kansasii
	M. fortuitum complex
	M. scrofulaceum (rarely)
Lymphadenitis (children)	M. scrofulaceum
	M. avium-intracellulare complex
Lymphadenitis (adults)	M. fortuitum complex
	M. avium-intracellulare complex
Swimming pool granuloma	M. marinum
"Sporotrichoid" lesions	M. marinum
	M. kansasii
Buruli ulcers with necrosis of fat	M. ulcerans
Postsurgical wound and percutaneous catheter infections	M. fortuitum complex
Cellulitis, abscesses	M. fortuitum complex
	M. avium-intracellulare complex
	M. kansasii
	M. ulcerans (rarely)
Disseminated cutaneous disease	M. avium-intracellulare complex
	M. fortuitum complex
	M. kansasii
	M. marinum (rarely)
	M. haemophilium
Reticuloendothelial dissemination	M. avium-intracellulare complex
	M. fortuitum complex
	M. kansasii
Bone and joint lesions	M. kansasii
	M. avium-intracellulare complex
	M. fortuitum complex
	M. marinum
Endocarditis	M. fortuitum complex
Keratitis, corneal ulcers	M. fortuitum complex

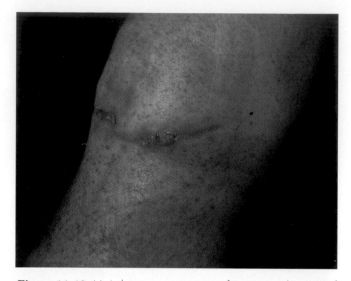

Figure 11.12 Mycobacterium marinum infection. Involvement of joint space with ulceration in scar secondary to knee surgery. (Courtesy of Dr. Lee T. Nesbitt, Jr.)

disease that may be much more difficult to clear. Disseminated infection to other areas of skin can occur in immunosuppressed patients (Figs. 11.14 and 11.15).

Mycobacterium kansasii is the nontuberculous organism most closely related to *M. tuberculosis*. Its natural habitat is unknown, but it has been found in tap water and both feral and domestic animals. The most common infection with this organism is pulmonary, usually in older patients with chronic lung disease. It may disseminate in patients who are immunosuppressed, producing skin lesions as well as involvement of lymph nodes, the musculoskeletal system, and other internal organs. Primary skin infections from *M. kansasii* are rare, usually being seen in immunosuppressed persons and occurring after cutaneous trauma.

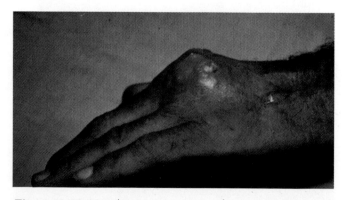

Figure 11.13 Mycobacterium marinum infection. Nodular lesion over joints of hand secondary to severe joint involvement and tenosynovitis. (Courtesy of Dr. Lee T. Nesbitt, Jr.)

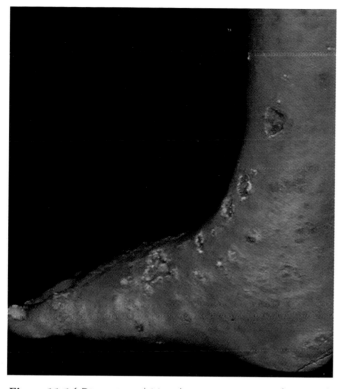

Figure 11.14 Disseminated *Mycobacterium marinum* infection. Ulcerative erythematous plaques with infiltration of skin of leg and foot in patient with Cushing's disease. (Courtesy of Dr. James Altick.)

Mycobacterium scrofulaceum is widely distributed and has been found in tap water, soil, and other sources in the environment. Infection usually occurs in young children, who become infected accidentally while playing. The portal of entry is usually by inhalation, with development of cervical lymphadenitis that later extends to form draining sinus tracts. The submandibular or submaxillary nodes are usually involved, rather than the

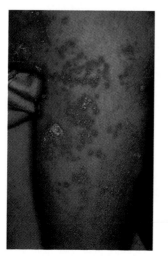

Figure 11.15 Disseminated *Mycobacterium marinum* infection. Widespread erythematous plaques on the leg of Cushing's disease patient shown in Figure 11.14. (Courtesy of Dr. James Altick.)

tonsillar and anterior cervical nodes characteristically involved in tuberculosis. No constitutional symptoms other than mild neck pain are present, and the disease is self-limited.

Mycobacterium avium and *Mycobacterium intracellulare* are closely related species that encompass over 20 subtypes. They can be found in many environmental sources including soil and water. The most common form of infection is pulmonary, and these infections are important in patients with acquired immunodeficiency syndrome (AIDS). Osteomyelitis and a cervical lymphadenitis with sinus formation are less common presentations of infection. Skin lesions are rare but may occur following traumatic inoculation.

Mycobacterium haemophilum produces cutaneous infections uncommonly, except in immunosuppressed individuals. Little is known about its natural habitat, although the organism has a propensity for growth in a cooler environment. When immunosuppressed patients develop disseminated lesions with acid-fast organisms that do not grow on standard Löwenstein-Jensen media, *M. haemophilum* infection should be considered. Cutaneous nodules or ulcerations are the usual lesions, either in localized or disseminated disease.

Mycobacterium ulcerans is most commonly found in tropical rain forests, especially in Africa. Most African cases occur on the extremities in children and young adults. The organism is introduced into the skin by a small puncture wound and produces a painless subcutaneous swelling after an incubation period of about 3 months. The nodule enlarges and ulcerates, producing an undermined lesion with discharge of necrotic fat. The ulceration eventually heals spontaneously. Scarring and lymphedema are common residual findings.

The *Mycobacterium fortuitum* complex includes *Mycobacterium chelonei*, the more common pathogen, and *M. fortuitum*. These organisms can be separated from other mycobacteria based on their rapid growth in culture. The organisms are widely distributed in nature and can be found in water and soil. Most cutaneous lesions have occurred postoperatively after mammoplasty, catheter placement, or other surgical procedures (Fig. 11.16). Another subset of infections occurs after traumatic abrasions in immunocompetent persons, and a final group of cutaneous lesions occurs in immunosuppressed patients with disseminated disease. The incubation period for cutaneous infection averages about 4 to 6 weeks. Local areas of cellulitis or abscess formation with sinus tract formation are presenting lesions. Disseminated disease can produce multiple soft tissue abscesses. The natural history of these lesions is chronic with slow healing, even with treatment. Spontaneous resolution occurs in a small percentage of patients.

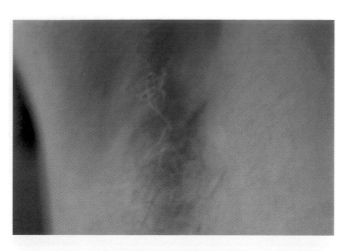

Figure 12.12 Axilla showing yellow colonies of trichomycosis on the hair shaft.

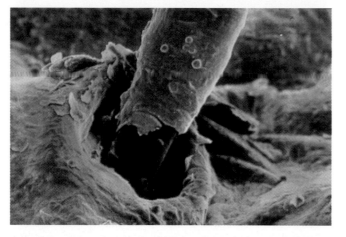

Figure 12.13 Scanning electron micrograph of colony on hair shaft in trichomycosis. (Copyright MediCire, London.)

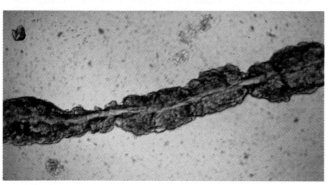

Figure 12.14 Squash preparation of coryneform colony from axillary hair from a patient with trichomycosis axillaris.

admixture of other genera cannot be excluded. Although there is damage to the hair visible by electron microscopy, the chief feature is the pronounced malodor that accompanies the microbial growth. This is ascribed to the modification of testosterone secreted by the apocrine glands to form a variety of compounds.[6] Unchecked eccrine sweating enables vigorous microbial growth to occur. Axillary malodor is most probably caused by a cocktail of compounds, and research in this area is far from complete. Diagnosis is made by visual and olfactory

means. Treatment is with topical antibacterials, or antibiotics may be used, but strict attention to hygiene and the use of axillary antiperspirants can also be effective. Undercutting of the axillary skin has been recommended as a more drastic solution to the problem of malodor.[7]

Normal Skin Inhabitants Among the other coryneform residents of normal human skin, two are associated with specific infections although others may appear in deep lesions of any tissue.

Corynebacterium jeikeium is a minor component of the skin flora, especially of males, that is found invading the bloodstream of patients receiving immunosuppressive therapy such as that prior to bone marrow transplantation for leukemia. About a quarter of such patients have concommitant skin or soft tissue infections with the same organism.[8] This species is usually resistant to many antibiotics, and therapy needs to be targeted with advice from the microbiology laboratory.

Members of the genus *Rhodococcus* are pathogens of animals; for example, *Rhodococcus equi* causes respiratory disease in foals.[9] Until relatively recently, *Rhodococcus* was difficult to differentiate from other coryneforms such as *Corynebacterium* or may have been included with the actinomycetes unless there was an index of suspicion, although a pale red pigment is produced on agar (Fig. 12.15). Prior to the advent of acquired immunodeficiency syndrome (AIDS), infection with *Rhodococcus* species was rare in humans, but this has changed. Skin disease has been reported in the immunocompetent on rare occasions, for example, a plaque-like cutaneous granuloma caused by *Rhodococcus rhodocrous* and a nodular lesion on the wrist of a child.[11] There are occasional reports of wound infection, but most infections in the immunodeficient patients are described as a slowly progressive pneumonia.[12] *Rhodococcus* isolates from human infections are frequently resistant to many antibiotics, and appropriate laboratory help should be sought.

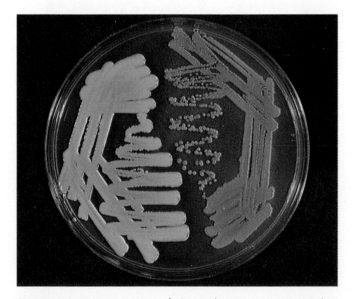

Figure 12.15 Comparison of *Corynebacterium* species (white colonies) and *Rhodococcus* species (pink colonies) on agar growth medium.

Propionibacterium *Species*

Three species of *Propionibacterium* are common inhabitants of human skin: *Propionibacterium acnes* and *Propionibacterium granulosum* (Fig. 12.16), which are found chiefly in the sebaceous areas, and *Propionibacterium avidum*, found chiefly in the axilla. A fourth species, *Propionibacterium propionicum*, is recovered from lachrymal gland infections and was formerly assigned to *Actinomyces* and then to *Arachnia*.[13] A minor component of the skin flora, *Propionibacterium innocuum*, has now been transferred to the new genus *Propioniferax* but is not associated with skin infection.

Acne Vulgaris   Acne occurs on the more sebaceous areas of the skin such as the chest and back, but particularly on the face, and may cause pitting on healing (Figs. 12.17 to 12.23). In patients with dark skin, pigmentation may make diagnosis more difficult by obscuring erythema. Although most frequent in teenage patients, acne does occur in other age groups. Males generally suffer more severe acne than females (Fig. 12.21). Acne is characterized by open comedones, frequently called blackheads from the abundant melanin at the skin surface, and by whitehead or closed comedones formed from swollen pilosebaceous ducts, which may become inflamed and pustular. There is now some doubt regarding the role of *P. acnes* and *P. granulosum* in acne. These organisms are probably not the cause of comedo formation but can be assigned a role in the inflammation that accompanies the lesions (Fig. 12.24). The normal site of growth of these bacteria is deep in the sebaceous follicles; when the sebum continues to be produced, organisms continue to grow, distending the follicle to form a closed comedone. Laboratory studies indicate that at extremely sharp pO$_2$ and pH optima, protease and hyaluronate lyase are produced; these would act to render the follicle wall permeable to the normal body defense mechanisms. Protease or the cell wall of *P. acnes* alone can activate the alternative complement pathway, initiating inflammation. A possible feedback loop is the action of porphyrins secreted by the *Propionibacterium* species in oxidizing squalene; squalene oxides may bring about changes in desquamation (Fig. 12.24).

Treatment of acne is dependent on the severity of disease. Mild disease can be treated with peeling agents to open the comedones; open comedones very rarely become inflamed. Topical or oral antibiotics form the next line of therapy, but it is worth noting that about one-third of patients who have received topical antibiotics now have *Propionibacterium* species resistant to those antibiotics. More aggressive therapies for severe disease (Fig. 12.22) include the retinoids and agents that alter hormonal balance.[14]

Figure 12.16 Propionibacterium acnes and Propionibacterium granulosum from lesion of acne. P. granulosum (the pink colonies) is almost always at a density 1/100 that of P. acnes.

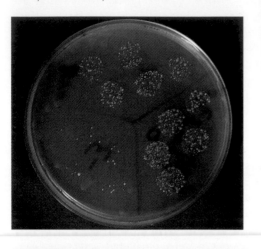

Figure 12.17 Typical acne lesions of the chest.

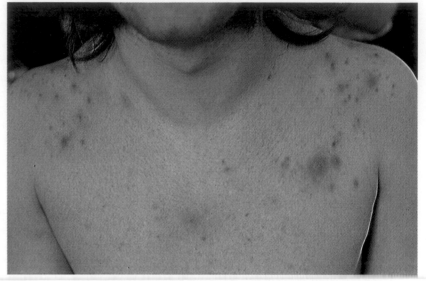

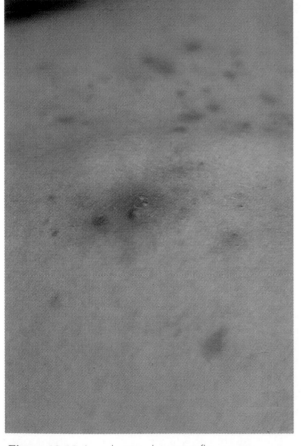

Figure 12.18 Acne lesions showing inflammation.

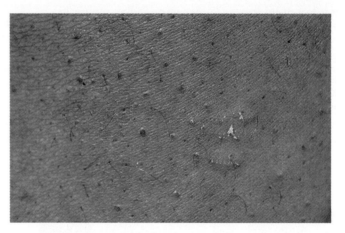

Figure 12.19 Acne in deeply pigmented skin. Erythema is much less obvious.

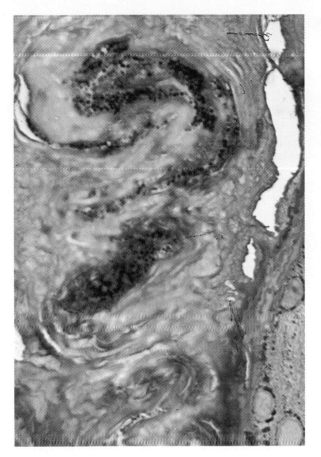

Figure 12.20 Microbial growth in distended follicle.

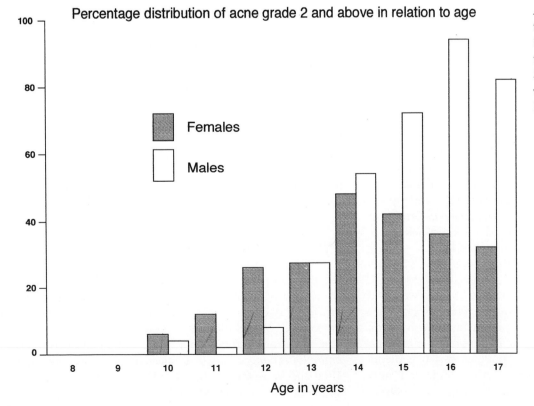

Percentage distribution of acne grade 2 and above in relation to age

Age in years

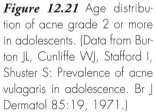

Figure 12.21 Age distribution of acne grade 2 or more in adolescents. (Data from Burton JL, Cunliffe WJ, Stafford I, Shuster S: Prevalence of acne vulagaris in adolescence. Br J Dermatol 85:19, 1971.)

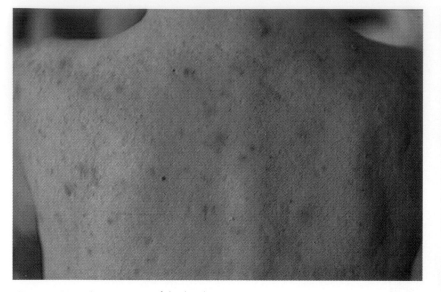

Figure 12.22 Severe acne of the back.

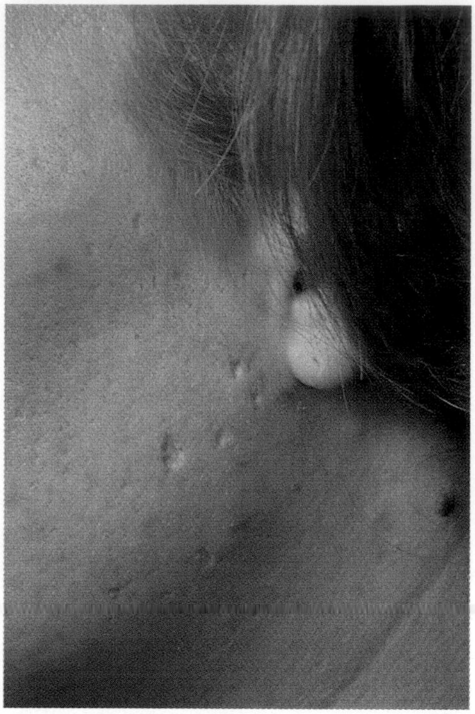

Figure 12.23 Pitting of skin due to acne scarring.

NONLIPOPHILIC OR LARGE-COLONY CORYNEFORMS

Brevibacterium *Species*

Members of the genus *Brevibacterium* were first recorded from human skin during a taxonomic study of cutaneous coryneforms; previously unidentified coryneform isolates from various infections of humans were then assigned to this genus, which had previously been confined to dairy specimens (*Brevibacterium linens*). A diagnostic feature was the evolution of the gas methane thiol, CH_3SH, which has a cheesy odor. The skin isolates were named *Brevibacterium epidermidis*, but this was followed by the recognition of other species including *Brevibacterium casei*. The majority of isolates from deep infections are *B. casei* and correspond to the Centers for Disease Control and Prevention (CDC) coryneform groups B1 and B3. But skin infections, usually of the feet, especially the toe webs and exhibiting severe erosions (Fig. 12.25), are weighted towards *B. epidermidis*; thus *Brevibacterium* species are responsible for the malodorous, nonitching erosive form of athlete's foot. A new species, *Brevibacterium mcbrellneri*, has been identified from nodules of white piedra from infected genital hair.[15] Further unnamed new species have been described from human feet. Occa-

sional deep infections such as a persistent bacteremia in an immunocompromised host have been reported.[16] Treatment with topical antibiotics is usually satisfactory, but the organisms are not susceptible to mupirocin. It is worth noting that topical antifungals such as miconazole also act against gram-positive bacteria.

Dermabacter *Species*

Dermabacter hominis is a nonlipophilic coryneform that forms a minor component of the normal skin flora that corresponds to the CDC fermentative groups 3 and 5. It has also been recovered from bloodstream and deep infections[17] but appears to play no part in cutaneous infection.

Pitted Keratolysis

Pitted keratolysis is associated with organisms that are not strictly coryneforms. The most consistent reports of the recovery of a specific organism from the crateriform pits on the soles of the feet that characterize this disease (Fig. 12.26) are of the actinomycete cattle pathogen *Dermatophilus congolensis*.[18] An alternative report concerns *Micrococcus sedentarius*.[19] Drying agents and topical antibiotics are usually satisfactory treatments.

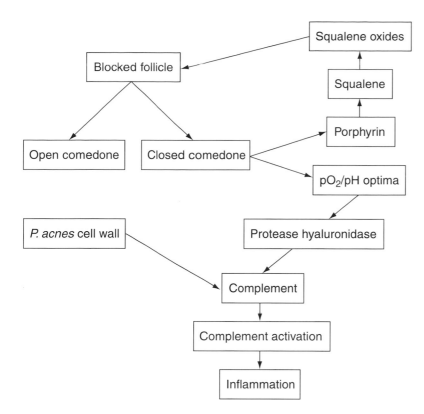

Figure 12.24 Schematic version of events that may result in inflammation of acne lesions.

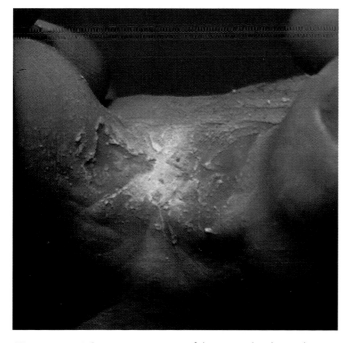

Figure 12.25 Severe maceration of the toe webs due to the protease activity of *Brevibacterium* species.

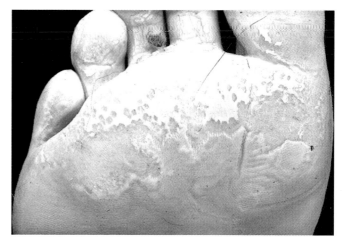

Figure 12.26 Pitted keratolysis, the result of proteolysis.

Figure 14.4 Nodular scabies on penis. (Courtesy of Dr. Axel W. Hoke.)

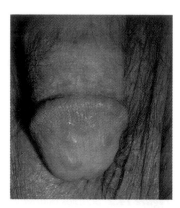

Figure 14.5 Scabies in an infant. Multiple burrows with pustules on soles. (Courtesy of Dr. Axel W. Hoke.)

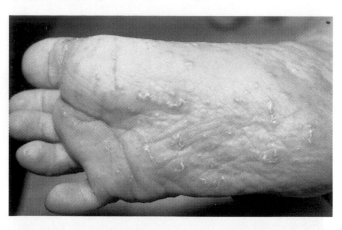

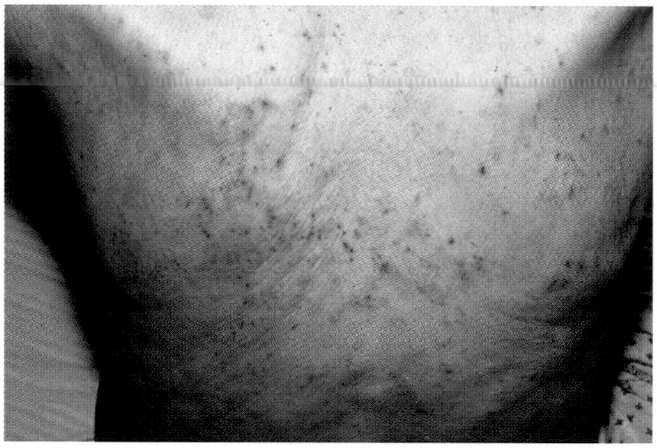

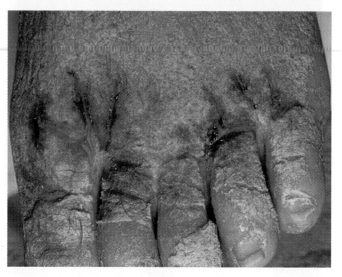

Figure 14.6 Scabies in the elderly. Numerous excoriations on the back.

Figure 14.7 Crusted scabies in AIDS. Diffuse involvement of top of foot. (Courtesy of Dr. Robert W. Goltz.)

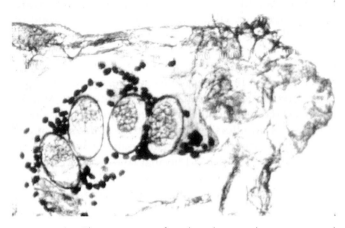

Figure 14.8 Skin scrapings of scabies burrow, large eggs, and numerous fecal pellets. (Courtesy of Dr. Axel W. Hoke.)

Complications

Secondary bacterial infection may occur. Nephritogenic streptococcal strains colonizing scabietic lesions and leading to acute glomerulonephritis have been reported, mainly in tropical areas, but the potential is universal. Eczema, particularly in atopic individuals, may be prominent in the active scabies infestation and may continue as eczema after the scabies is cleared.

Acarophobia (or the more inclusive term, "delusions of parasitosis") may occur in individuals who have been successfully treated for scabies or never had scabies; treatment for these patients is extremely difficult.

Treatment

Principles The choice of drug should be based on efficacy and potential toxicity (Table 14.1). Patients often apply medications more frequently and over longer periods than prescribed. Limiting the quantity prescribed prevents dermatitis caused by overtreatment, which the patient may mistake for the persistence of scabies. Treatment is preceded by a tepid bath or shower and then drying with a towel. Scabicides should be applied thinly but thoroughly to the area behind the ears from the neck down to all areas, with special attention to the areas between the fingers, the umbilical area, the groin, between the buttocks, between the toes, and particularly under the fingernails and toenails, which should be trimmed short. Medication should be left on for the number of hours suggested, then thoroughly rinsed off with tepid water and the skin dried. At the conclusion of therapy, intimate articles of clothing, bed linens, and towels should be machine washed and dried, using the hot cycle of each machine.

Selected treatment of asymptomatic family members at high risk for acquiring the infestation from a confirmed case is appropriate (e.g., if the patient shares a bed with another person, sexual contact).

Table 14.1 Treatment of Scabies

TREATMENT	OUR USE	HOW TO USE	TOXICITY	TOLERANCE (RESISTANCE)	ACCEPTANCE	COST
Permethrin cream 5%	Do not use in infants < 2 mo of age, pregnant and lactating women, hypersensitivity	10 h × 1[a]	Low	None	Aesthetic	Higher
Lindane lotion 1%	Do not use in infants or small children, pregnant or lactating women, significant neurologic disease, hypersensitivity	8 h × 1[a]	Possible CNS	Alleged	Aesthetic	Lower
Precipitated sulfur unguent 6%	Infants < 2 mo of age, pregnant and lactating women	24-h periods at night × 3	Low	None	Messy	Pharmacist compounded

[a] There are no controlled studies that document that two applications are better than one. May repeat in 1 week if there is microscopic and/or morphologic evidence of treatment failure.

Another form of cutaneous infection caused by HSV-1 occurs among wrestlers (herpes gladiatorum) and rugby players ("scrum-pox").[11,12] Infection results from close contact between abraded skin and oral secretions. Any damaged area of skin is susceptible to direct inoculation of HSV. For example, severe diaper dermatitis, burned skin, or skin affected by atopic dermatitis is susceptible to severe infection following autoinoculation of HSV-1 or transmission during close contact from an active oral lesion of a caretaker.[13] Another cutaneous complication of HSV is precipitation of erythema multiforme; skin biopsies from 12 of 16 patients with erythema multiforme were positive for an HSV antigen in one study.[14]

Neonatal Infection

Most neonates infected with HSV contract the virus at delivery (perinatal infection). However, about 5% of infected neonates acquire infection in utero and have true congenital infection. Manifestations of congenital infection include abnormalities of the skin, eye, and brain. Skin abnormalities include extensive vesicles or bullae or scars involving the scalp, face, trunk, or extremities. Eye abnormalities include keratoconjunctivitis, chorioretinitis, and microphthalmia, and central nervous system (CNS) abnormalities include microcephaly and hydranencephaly. The largest experience with intrauterine HSV infections included 13 babies. The relative frequency of findings among these 13 babies included some combination of skin lesions and scars (12), chorioretinitis (8), microcephaly (7), hydranencephaly (5), and microphthalmia (2).[15]

Neonates perinatally infected with HSV almost always develop signs of infection by 4 to 5 weeks of age (Fig. 15.4 to 15.9). Infection is classified according to whether it is localized or disseminated. Localized infection may involve the skin, eye, and mouth or the CNS. Infection localized to the skin, eye, and mouth accounts for about 40% of all neonatal HSV infections, whereas 35% of infections are localized to the CNS, and 25% are disseminated.[16] Although this general classification is useful, there is considerable overlap between the different forms of infection. For example, neonates with CNS or disseminated infection may develop skin or mucosal lesions diagnostic of HSV infection.

The skin, eye, and mouth form of neonatal HSV infection has the most favorable prognosis if diagnosis and appropriate antiviral therapy are prompt. In the absence of therapy, about 75% of cases of neonatal skin, eye, and mouth infection progress to disseminated or CNS disease.[17]

Neonates with disseminated HSV infection typically develop signs of infection during the first several days of life. Common clinical findings include vascular instability, hepatosplenomegaly, jaundice, and respiratory dysfunction. Their illness is often confused with overwhelming bacterial infection. Although almost three-quarters of patients develop mucocutaneous findings typical of HSV, lesions often are absent at the onset of symptoms. Infection progresses rapidly, and more than 70% of untreated neonates die as a result of unremitting shock, progressive liver dysfunction with widespread bleeding, respiratory failure, or progressive neurologic dysfunction.[17]

The form of neonatal HSV infection that presents latest in life is CNS disease. Signs and symptoms of encephalitis usually appear between 2 and 3 weeks of age. Fever and lethargy are followed by seizures, which tend to be focal and difficult to control. Skin lesions are present in nearly half of infected infants at presentation. Cerebrospinal fluid analysis is typical of any other viral meningoencephalitis, with less than 100 white blood cells/mm^3 (predominantly mononuclear) and normal or slightly reduced glucose concentration. However, cerebrospinal fluid protein concentration tends to be more markedly elevated (as high as 500 to 1,000 mg/dl) than that of other encephalitides. The electroencephalogram usually is diffusely abnormal. Although computed axial tomography of the head often is normal early in the course of infection, magnetic resonance imaging usually is abnormal.

DIAGNOSIS

Viral Isolation

The most sensitive method for diagnosing HSV infection is viral isolation. The highest yield of cultures is from mucocutaneous lesions. Timing of specimen collection is critical. For example, HSV is recovered from more than 90% of genital herpes lesions cultured during the vesicular stage but less than 30% during the crusted stage.[18] The optimal technique for sampling intact lesions is to aspirate their contents with a small sterile needle. Alternatively, samples can be obtained by unroofing vesicles with a sterile needle and vigorously swabbing their bases with premoistened sterile cotton-tipped swabs. Calcium alginate swabs should not be used, as they inhibit viral growth.[19] Ideally, specimens should be directly inoculated into 1 to 2 ml of viral transport media and transported to the diagnostic laboratory. If storage of specimens prior to transport is necessary, they should be maintained at −70°C; freezing at −20°C before processing reduces viability of HSV.

In some clinical situations, such as suspected neonatal herpes, tissue culture isolation of HSV is too slow, and more rapid diagnostic tests also should be utilized. The

Figure 15.5 Neonatal HSV infection.

Figure 15.4 Neonatal HSV infection.

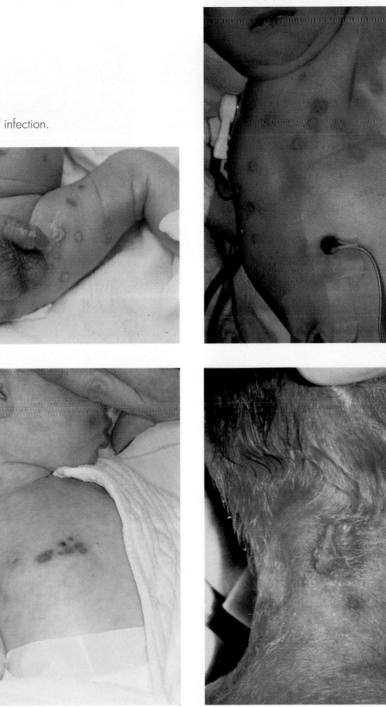

Figure 15.6 Neonatal HSV infection.

Figure 15.7 Neonatal HSV infection.

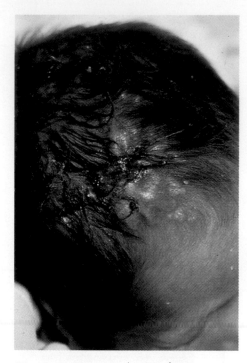

Figure 15.8 Neonatal HSV infection.

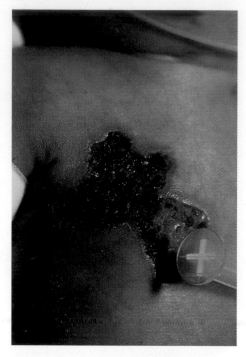

Figure 15.9 Neonatal HSV infection.

most commonly used rapid diagnostic test useful for the evaluation of mucocutaneous lesions is direct immunofluorescent staining.[20] This test is performed on specimens obtained by unroofing lesions, vigorously swabbing their bases with the blunt end of cotton applicator sticks, and streaking the collected material onto glass slides. Direct staining of samples with fluorescein-conjugated monoclonal HSV antibodies has a sensitivity compared to tissue culture of 80 to 90%, and there are few false-positive reactions. Although the Papanicolaou stain or Tzanck test can be used to demonstrate cytologic changes in specimens obtained from suspected HSV lesions, their sensitivity is limited and their use discouraged.[21] The typical histologic appearance of cutaneous HSV lesions is illustrated in Figures 15.10 and 15.11.

Serology

There are a number of commercially available serologic tests able to detect the presence of HSV IgG antibodies. However, because of extensive antigenic homology between HSV-1 and HSV-2, these assays cannot reliably differentiate between HSV-1 and HSV-2 antibodies.

TREATMENT

Acyclovir is the drug of choice for most HSV infections. Available formulations include topical ointment, oral tablets, liquid, and a preparation for intravenous use (Table 15.2).

Orolabial Infection

Systemic acyclovir should be effective for the therapy of primary HSV gingivostomatitis. It is more active in vitro against HSV-1 than HSV-2, and results of a placebo-controlled trial in children with primary gingivostomatitis were encouraging.[22] It is reasonable to treat patients with parenteral acyclovir if they have moderate or severe primary oral herpes infections, especially if they are hospitalized to receive intravenous fluid support. The role of acyclovir in the therapy of recurrent oral herpes infections is not clear. Even when administered immediately after the onset of symptoms, neither topical nor oral acyclovir offers substantial clinical benefit to immunocompetent hosts with recurrent labial infections.[23,24] However, prophylactically administered oral acyclovir may be useful in selected individuals with frequently recurrent oral infections. Compared with placebo, acyclovir resulted in a greater than 50% reduction in clinical recurrences among 56 adults who prior to treatment had six or more recurrent episodes of herpes labialis per year.[25] Prophylactically administered oral acyclovir also reduces the risk or severity of oral herpes outbreaks among patients prone to recurrences as a result of trigeminal ganglion surgery, ultraviolet light exposure, or alpine skiing.[26–28]

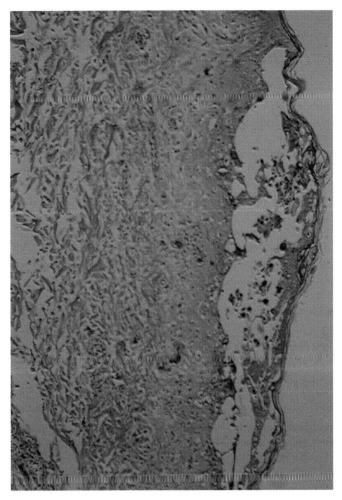

Figure 15.10 Histologic views of cutaneous lesions.

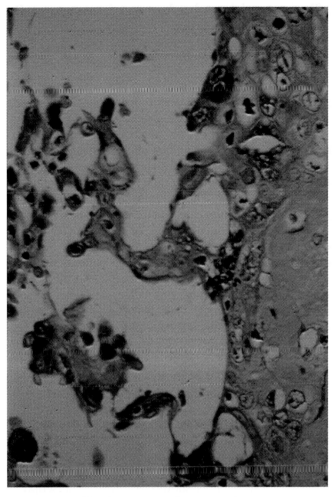

Figure 15.11 Histologic views of cutaneous lesions.

Table 15.2 Therapy of Mucocutaneous HSV Infections

INFECTION	RECOMMENDED THERAPY	ANTICIPATED BENEFITS
Initial genital herpes	Oral acyclovir, 40 mg/kg/day in 4 doses for 5–10 days	3- to 12-day reduction in duration of viral shedding and time to healing, and 1–10 day reduction in duration of pain
Recurrent genital herpes	Oral acyclovir, 40 mg/kg/day in 4 divided doses for 5–10 days	1- to 2-day reduction in duration of viral shedding and time to healing; no difference in duration of pain
Primary herpes labialis (HSV gingivostomatitis)	Oral acyclovir, 40 mg/kg/day in 4 divided doses for 5–10 days	6-day reduction in duration of viral shedding and 2- to 4-day reduction in duration of drooling, gum swelling, and healing of oral and cutaneous lesions
Recurrent herpes labialis	Oral acyclovir, 40 mg/kg/day in 4 divided doses for 5–10 days	1- to 2-day reduction in duration of pain and time to healing
Mucocutaneous HSV infections in compromised hosts	IV acyclovir, 15 mg/kg/day in 3 divided doses for 7–10 days	60–80% reduction in duration of viral shedding, 30–60% reduction in healing time and duration in pain
Neonatal HSV infections	IV acyclovir, 60 mg/kg/day in 3 divided doses for 14–21 days	Reduced mortality and improved long-term outcome

(Data from Spruance et al.,[23] Stone and Whittington,[29] Whitley et al.,[31] Straus et al.,[32] and Whitley.[33])

Figure 16.5 Herpes zoster. Grouped vesicopustules on erythematous bases on the trunk. (Courtesy of Dr. Lee T. Nesbitt, Jr.)

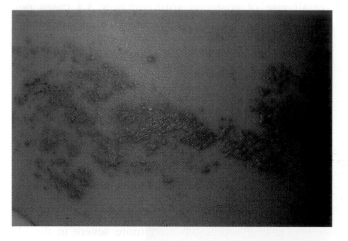

Figure 16.6 Herpes zoster. Grouped vesicopustules on erythematous bases on the back, showing lesions extending to the midline. (Courtesy of Dr. Lee T. Nesbitt, Jr.)

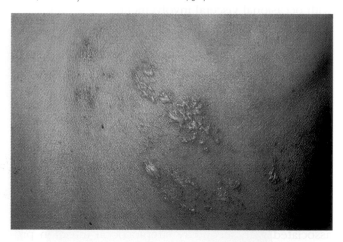

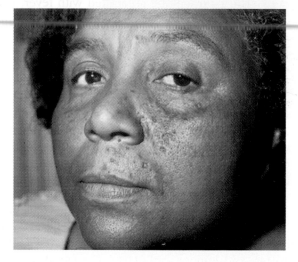

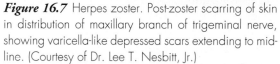

Figure 16.7 Herpes zoster. Post-zoster scarring of skin in distribution of maxillary branch of trigeminal nerve, showing varicella-like depressed scars extending to midline. (Courtesy of Dr. Lee T. Nesbitt, Jr.)

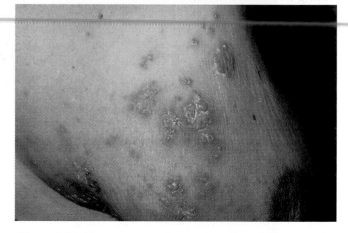

Figure 16.8 Herpes zoster. Grouped vesicopustules on erythematous bases on the breast, showing lesions with necrosis beneath the breast. (Courtesy of Dr. Lee T. Nesbitt, Jr.)

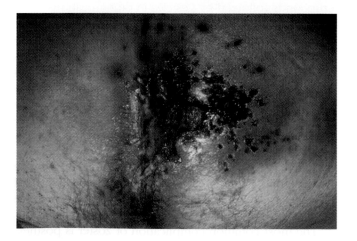

Figure 16.9 Herpes zoster. Gangrenous, necrotic lesions of buttocks extending to midline. (Courtesy of Dr. Lee T. Nesbitt, Jr.)

Figure 16.10 Herpes zoster. Bullous lesions of forehead in a child extending to midline, in distribution of ophthalmic branch of trigeminal nerve. (Courtesy of Dr. Lee T. Nesbitt, Jr.)

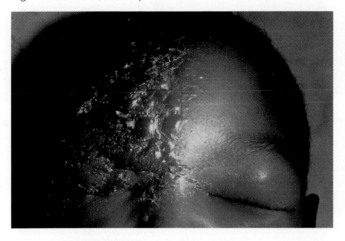

Figure 16.11 Herpes zoster. Grouped vesicles on erythematous bases with one necrotic area near angle of mouth; lesions are in distribution of mandibular branch of trigeminal nerve and simulate herpes simplex. (Courtesy of Dr. Lee T. Nesbitt, Jr.)

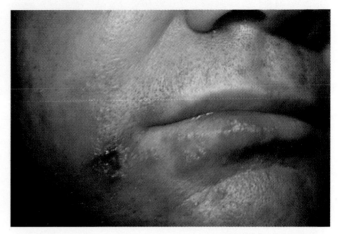

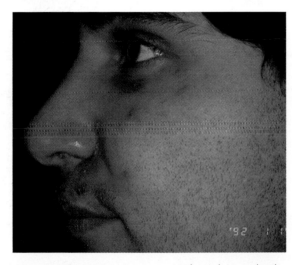

Figure 16.12 Herpes zoster. Unilateral vesicular lesions in distribution of maxillary branch of trigeminal nerve. (Courtesy of Dr. Lee T. Nesbitt, Jr.)

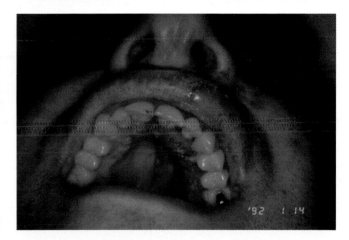

Figure 16.13 Herpes zoster. Unilateral necrotic lesions of oral mucosa and skin extending to midline, in distribution of maxillary branch of trigeminal nerve. Same patient as in Figure 16.12. (Courtesy of Dr. Lee T. Nesbitt, Jr.)

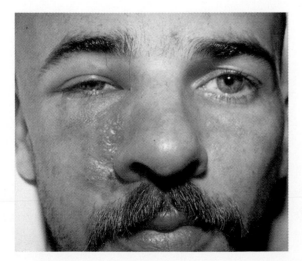

Figure 16.14 Herpes zoster. Unilateral erythema and edema with early vesicular lesions in a human immunodeficiency virus (HIV)–positive patient, in distribution of maxillary branch of trigeminal nerve. (Courtesy of Dr. Lee T. Nesbitt, Jr.)

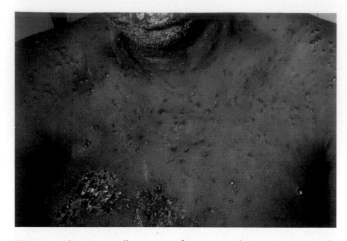

Figure 16.15 Varicella-zoster infection. Leukemic patient with herpes zoster of chest and generalized vesicular eruption. (Courtesy of Dr. Lee T. Nesbitt, Jr.)

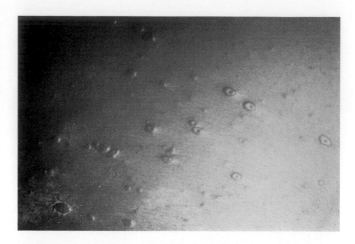

Figure 16.16 Varicella-zoster infection. Vesicular lesions of trunk, some with central umbilication. Same patient as in Figure 16.15. (Courtesy of Dr. Lee T. Nesbitt, Jr.)

petic neuralgia, occurring in about 15% of cases. Over half of patients over age 60 experiencing zoster have pain greater than 1 month after resolution of lesions. Half of these are pain free at 3 months. Most patients report a marked decrease in pain by 6 months, but the duration and severity are variable. Postherpetic neuralgia is most common after cases of ophthalmic zoster.[1]

Involvement of the central nervous system should be suspected in cases of zoster associated with headache. The complications include encephalitis, peripheral motor neuropathies, cranial nerve palsies, optic neuritis, myelitis, thrombotic vasculopathy, and Ramsay Hunt syndrome with hearing loss and tinnitus.[6]

Ocular complications can occur in many cases of ophthalmic zoster (Fig. 16.17); these especially are seen when the cutaneous eruption involves the tip of the nose, indicating involvement of the nasociliary nerve. The conjunctiva is often red and swollen, and keratitis of variable severity may develop. Other complications include cicatricial lid retraction, ptosis, Argyll Robertson pupil, glaucoma, retinitis, choroiditis, optic neuritis, optic atrophy, retrobulbar neuritis, exophthalmos, and extraocular muscle palsies. Ocular disease associated with VZV may rarely occur in the absence of skin involvement.[5]

In immunosuppressed patients, zoster frequently re-

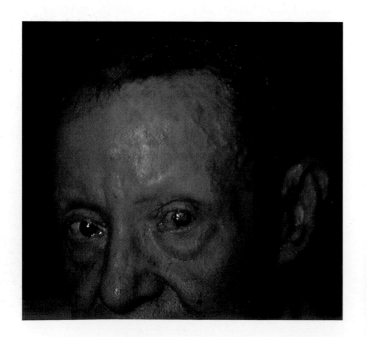

Figure 16.17 Herpes zoster. Post-zoster scarring of skin and eye, in distribution of ophthalmic branch of trigeminal nerve. (Courtesy of Dr. Lee T. Nesbitt, Jr.)

sults in disseminated disease with visceral involvement. Progressive outer retinal necrosis is a VZV-mediated disease associated with low CD4 counts in patients with acquired immunodeficiency syndrome (AIDS), the disease is generally rapidly progressive to blindness despite antiviral therapy.[7] Persistent localized disease includes the chronic verrucous zoster lesions seen in AIDS patients and the chronic ecthymatous nodules described in patients with cutaneous T-cell lymphoma.[8]

PATHOLOGY

Primary varicella is usually acquired by direct inhalation of infectious material but can be acquired by contact with skin lesions. After the initial infection of respiratory mucosa, the virus replicates within regional lymph nodes before the primary viremia occurs. After replication in the liver and spleen, a second viremia results in spread to the skin.

The infected epithelial cells undergo ballooning degeneration (Fig. 16.18) with eosinophilic Cowdry type I intranuclear inclusion bodies. Some epidermal cells fuse via viral glycoproteins to produce multinucleate cells. The epithelial degeneration and edema produce vesicles with large amounts of infectious virions.

The mechanisms involved in zoster are not completely understood, but it is thought that during the course of varicella, virus spreads from the epidermis to cutaneous sensory nerves and travels along the nerve fibers to dorsal ganglion cells. There the virus persists for an extended period without obvious clinical activity. The dorsal ganglia most often involved parallel the anatomic sites with the highest concentration of cutaneous lesions.

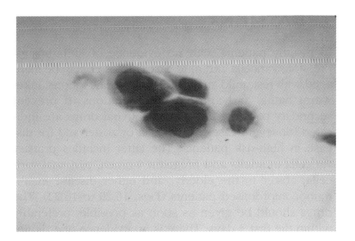

Figure 16.19 Herpesvirus infection. Multinucleate giant cell on smear from base of vesicular lesion (Tzanck preparation). (Courtesy of Dr. Lee T. Nesbitt, Jr.)

Subclinical reactivation probably occurs at various intervals and may boost levels of immunity. At a later time of depressed cellular immunity from various factors or the natural decline in cellular immunity associated with aging, the virus reactivates, replicates within the ganglion, spreads down the nerve causing radiculoneuritis, and is released into the skin around nerve endings. The histologic findings are identical to those in primary varicella.[1]

DIAGNOSIS

To confirm the clinical diagnosis of VZV infection, a variety of laboratory tests can be utilized. The Tzanck smear (Fig. 16.19) is obtained by scraping the base of an early vesicular lesion and staining the smear with one of various stains, such as Wright's stain. The presence of multinucleate cells and viral inclusions indicates a herpesvirus but is unable to distinguish VZV from herpes simplex virus. Tissue histopathology and electron microscopy have similar limitations. Historically, culture has been the usual method to differentiate these viruses, but it is hampered by the fact that VZV is only cultured in about 70% of cases and requires 7 to 21 days to grow. The direct fluorescent antibody technique has many advantages over culture, as it is more sensitive, less expensive, and faster.[9] Polymerase chain reaction is even more sensitive and rapidly demonstrates small amounts of viral DNA in biopsies of skin lesions, peripheral mononuclear cells, CSF, or other tissues. Serologic tests are used primarily to determine immune status, but serology utilizing complement fixation can also be used in CSF to look for evidence of recent infection.

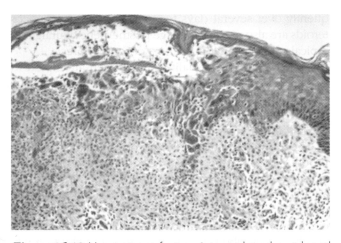

Figure 16.18 Herpesvirus infection. Intraepidermal vesicle with ballooning degeneration of epidermal cells and formation of multinucleate giant cells. (Courtesy of Dr. Carmen G. Espinoza.)

munization include fever, pain at the injection site within the first 48 hours, a low incidence of a varicella-like rash at the injection site, and a low incidence of a mild generalized varicella-like eruption. Adults usually require two doses for optimal seroconversion; they also exhibit lower cell-mediated and humoral immune response and experience more frequent breakthrough disease.[14] The elderly commonly experience attenuated responses to the vaccine, with about 10 to 15% of vaccinees failing to exhibit any boost in immunity regardless of the vaccine dose.[15] Booster doses can be administered to individuals who have preexisting immunity with no greater risks than to nonimmune individuals. Since zoster is hypothesized to occur because of the gradual decline in VZV-specific cell-mediated immunity related to aging, it is thought that the vaccine may provide a way of stimulating cellular immunity to the virus and preventing zoster. The few cases of zoster in children after immunization argue against this concept, but it remains to be seen what the outcome will be in various populations receiving the vaccine with boosters.

Children receiving chemotherapy for lymphoproliferative disease can be successfully vaccinated for VZV. It is recommended that chemotherapy be suspended for a week before and after immunization. Half the children with acute myelogenous leukemia receiving maintenance chemotherapy or corticosteroids will experience a mild maculopapular or vesicular rash within a month of vaccination. There is a 20 to 25% risk of transmission of vaccine-type virus from leukemia vaccinees to nonimmune household contacts, but the disease is usually mild.

DIFFERENTIAL DIAGNOSIS

Since varicella is a widespread eruption, its differential diagnosis is more extensive than that of zoster. Lesions of varicella must be differentiated from arthropod bites, scabies, erythema multiforme, other viral exanthems, drug eruptions, histiocytosis X, pityriasis lichenoides, and dermatitis herpetiformis. Usually the dermatomal distribution of zoster makes clinical diagnosis apparent, but the differential diagnosis includes contact dermatitis, arthropod bites, bacterial infections, other viral infections, and burns. Herpes simplex (Fig. 16.23) can be especially difficult to differentiate, as it may present with a dermatomal vesicular eruption similar to zoster; a recurrent eruption should particularly lead to consideration of herpes simplex virus as the likely culprit (Fig. 16.24). Since pain frequently precedes the eruption, many erroneous diagnoses may be made such as herniated intervertebral disk, pleurisy, myocardial infarction, cholecystitis, acute odontalgia, appendicitis, ovarian cyst, duodenal ulcer, fracture, tendinitis, or renal calculus. When zoster occurs without a rash, the diagnosis is particularly difficult. In these cases, the diagnosis hinges on serologic tests, histopathology, or polymerase chain reaction.

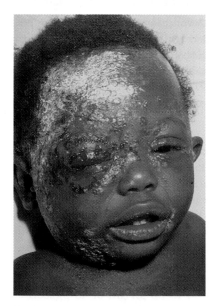

Figure 16.23 Primary herpes simplex infection. Numerous vesicles, crusts, and erosions extending across the midline of face in a child. Differential diagnosis includes varicella-zoster infection. (Courtesy of Dr. Lee T. Nesbitt, Jr.)

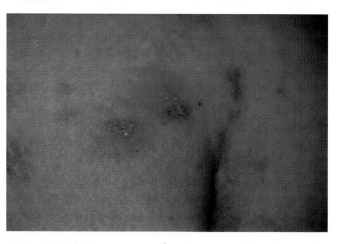

Figure 16.24 Recurrent zosteriform herpes simplex infection. Recurrent grouped vesicular lesions on erythematous bases with scarring of the buttocks in a female patient. Differential diagnosis includes herpes zoster. (Courtesy of Dr. Lee T. Nesbitt, Jr.)

REFERENCES

1. Rockley PF, Tyring SK: Pathophysiology and clinical manifestations of varicella zoster virus infections. Int J Dermatol 33:227, 1994

2. Junker AK, Tilley P: Varicella-zoster virus antibody avidity and IgG-subclass patterns in children with recurrent chickenpox. J Med Virol 43:119, 1994

3. Enders G. Consequences of varicella and herpes zoster in pregnancy: prospective study of 1739 cases. Lancet 343:1548, 1994

4. Doctor A et al: Group A beta-hemolytic streptococcal bacteremia: historical overview, changing incidence, and recent association with varicella. Pediatrics 96:428, 1995

5. Highet AS, Kurtz J: Varicella (chickenpox) and zoster (shingles). p. 885. In Champion RN, Burton JL, Ebling FJG (eds): Textbook of Dermatology. 5th Ed. Vol 2. Blackwell Scientific Publications, London, 1992

6. Elliot KJ: Other neurological complications of herpes zoster and their management. Ann Neurol suppl. 35:S57, 1994

7. Greven CM et al: Progressive outer retinal necrosis secondary to varicella zoster virus in acquired immune deficiency syndrome. Retina 15:14, 1995

8. Erhard H et al: Atypical varicella-zoster virus infection in an immunocompromised patient: result of a virus-induced vasculitis. J Am Acad Dermatol 32:908, 1995

9. Zirn JR et al: Rapid detection and distinction of cutaneous herpesvirus infections by direct immunofluorescence. J Am Acad Dermatol 33:724, 1995

10. Nikkels AF, Pierard GE: Recognition and treatment of shingles. Drugs 48:528, 1994

11. Watson CPN: The treatment of postherpetic neuralgia. Neurology 45, suppl. 8:S58, 1995

12. Clements DA et al: Over five-year follow-up of Oka/Merck varicella vaccine recipients in 465 infants and adolescents. Pediatr Infect Dis J 14:874, 1995

13. Matsubara K et al: Herpes zoster in a normal child after varicella vaccination. Acta Paediatr Jpn 37:648, 1995

14. Nader S et al: Age-related differences in cell-mediated immunity to varicella-zoster virus among children and adults immunized with live attenuated varicella vaccine. J Infect Dis 171:13, 1995

15. Levin MJ et al: Immune responses of elderly persons 4 years after receiving a live attenuated varicella vaccine. J Infect Dis 170:522, 1994

CHAPTER 17

Skin Infections in the Immunocompromised Patient

Timothy G. Berger

SUMMARY

Etiology   Viruses, bacteria, and fungi

Clinical Features   Mucocutaneous infection, genital infection, cutaneous infection, orbital infection

Diagnosis   Skin biopsy, cultures

Treatment   Antiviral therapy, antibacterial, antifungal

Differential Diagnosis   See sections for individual infections

Organ transplantation, aggressive management of malignancy with chemotherapy and bone marrow transplantation, the survival of very low birth weight infants, and the human immunodeficiency virus (HIV) epidemic have made immunosuppressed patients common in clinical practice. These forms of immunosuppression have shown us that it is no longer possible to lump all immunosuppressed hosts together. While certain infectious agents are a particular burden for many immunosuppressed hosts, clinical patterns differ in patients with the various forms of immunosuppression. Cutaneous cryptococcosis often presents as cellulitis in the organ transplant patient with iatrogenic immunosuppression; this pattern is not reported in the acquired immunodeficiency syndrome (AIDS) patient, in whom it presents as papules resembling molluscum contagiosum. Neutropenia specifically is a risk factor for systemic candidiasis, aspergillosis, and Pseudomonas sepsis, independent of the underlying disease leading to granulocytopenia. The fact that the patient is immunosuppressed should alert the clinician to the possibility of an unusual pathogen or clinical presentation, and the specific form of immunosuppression may also predict the infectious agents to which the patient is predisposed.

In the immunocompetent patient, the general rule of "One patient, one diagnosis" applies. In immunosuppression, especially in the setting of HIV disease, combinations of infections are not uncommon. *Staphylococcus aureus* may infect lesions due to herpes simplex virus (HSV), which may be seen in the genital area in association with human papillomavirus infection. Atypical mycobacteria and systemic fungal infection may be identified in skin lesions due primarily to other agents such as HSV.

S. aureus and streptococci are common pathogens in immunosuppressed hosts. Folliculitis, abscesses, and cellulitis all occur. Neutropenia and the presence of an indwelling central line may be additional risk factors for the development of sepsis (Fig. 17.1).

Pseudomonas aeruginosa causes skin lesions with extensive cutaneous necrosis (ecthyma gangrenosum) (Fig. 17.2). Lesions favor the apocrine areas, especially the groin. Ecthyma gangrenosum was originally thought to be specifically associated with *Pseudomonas* sepsis, but it also occurs in the absence of sepsis.[1,2] Neutropenia is the major risk factor for the development of ecthyma gangrenosum, with or without sepsis; consequently this complication is most frequently seen in patients with myelodysplastic disorders. The treatment of *Pseudomonas* infection in the immunosuppressed host is intravenous antibiotics to which the organism is sensitive. Oral quinolones may be used to complete therapy if appropriate.

Bartonella henselae (the cat-scratch disease bacillus) and *Bartonella quintana* (the cause of trench fever) are important pathogens in HIV-infected patients, especially those with T-helper cell counts below 200 mm³. The clinical features of infection with these two organisms are identical. Blood-borne infection occurs, sometimes without systemic symptoms (analogous to household cats who are frequently bacteremic with *B. henselae* but appear totally well). Skin lesions are frequently observed, presenting most commonly as fleshy, angiomatous papules resembling pyogenic granulomas (Fig. 17.3). This pattern of disease has been called bacillary angiomatosis. Dermal or subcutaneous papules, cellulitic plaques, and large tumors or ulcerations are other cutaneous presentations (Fig. 17.4). Apparently the organ-

Figure 17.1 Purpuric plaques of acute onset in a neutropenic patient with leukemia. Blood and skin cultures grew *Staphylococcus aureus*.

Figure 17.2 Ecthyma gangrenosum. Purpuric plaque on the leg in a neutropenic patient associated with *Pseudomonas* sepsis.

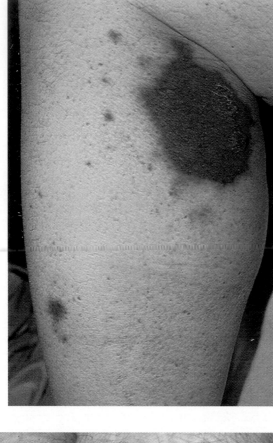

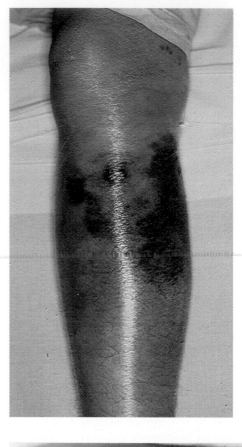

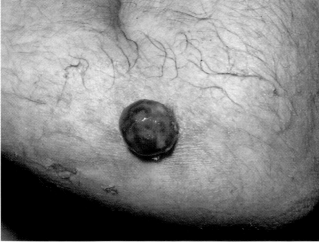

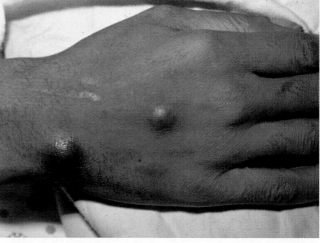

Figure 17.3 Bacillary angiomatosis. Friable, pyogenic granuloma-like nodule in an AIDS patient.

Figure 17.4 Bacillary angiomatosis. Subcutaneous nodules in a febrile AIDS patient. Both *Mycobacterium avium-intracellulare* (MAC) and *Bartonella* species were identified in the lesion. The nodules resolved with therapy directed only at *Bartonella* species suggesting the MAC was not primarily pathogenic.

isms are introduced through the skin (as in cat-scratch disease), and patients may report that lesions appeared at sites of such trauma. Over time, in the untreated patient, the number of lesions increases, and the individual lesions appear more miliary. Infection may involve other organ systems, including (in decreasing order of apparent frequency) lymphatics, liver and spleen, bone, muscle (pyomyositis), pulmonary system, and central nervous system.

The diagnosis of *Bartonella* infection is difficult, since routine laboratory culture methods may not isolate the causative bacilli. Skin lesions are an excellent source of diagnostic material. Typical histologic features in combination with identification of the organisms by silver stains or electron microscopy are the currently applied methods. Polymerase chain reaction can be used to identify this infection in atypical or paucibacillary cases. In the immunosuppressed host, infections with *Bartonella* species should be treated with a minimum of 8 weeks of antibiotics, with 2g of erythromycin or 200 mg of doxycycline daily having been used most extensively. Documented visceral disease (liver, spleen, bone) may require longer courses of therapy (4 to 6 months).

Nocardia species are gram-positive filamentous rods. They infect both immunosuppressed and immunocompetent hosts. *Nocardia asteroides* is the most common species isolated, but *Nocardia brasiliensis* and *Nocardia caviae* may also cause human disease. Thirteen percent of all cases of nocardial infection occur in transplant patients, with about 13% of cardiac transplant patients and 1 to 20% of renal transplant patients developing infection, often long after transplantation.[3,4] Pulmonary infection is the most common form. About 5% of all cases of nocardiosis are primary cutaneous infections (direct inoculation), but skin lesions may also occur by hematogenous spread from a visceral focus. The clinical features of primary cutaneous nocardiosis and hematogenous cutaneous infection may be similar. Clinical forms of skin infection include lymphocutaneous (sporotricoid); abscesses, pustules, ulcers, cellulitis; and mycetoma.

The diagnosis of nocardiosis is confirmed by culture but should be suspected if the typical gram-positive, weakly acid-fast branching filamentous organisms are seen in clinical material. Sulfonamides alone or in combination with trimethoprim are the treatment of choice. Minocycline and ampicillin (with or without clavulanic acid) are available oral alternatives to which the majority of clinical *Nocardia* isolates are sensitive. Prolonged therapy seems to be the key to management, rather than combination antibiotic therapy. Immunosuppressive medications usually do not need to be discontinued or reduced for therapeutic success.

ACID-FAST BACILLI

HIV infection and increasing immigration from countries where tuberculosis is common have led to an increase in tuberculosis in the developed world. Immunosuppressed patients may rarely develop cutaneous lesions as a complication of reactivating their pulmonary tuberculosis. In the developed countries, the most common skin lesions seen in HIV-infected patients (other than scrofuloderma) are those of disseminated miliary tuberculosis (Fig. 17.5). These appear as small hemorrhagic or brown papules or papulopustules.[5] Biopsy shows acute neutrophilic inflammation without granulomas but with numerous acid-fast bacilli. Tuberculous abscesses and miliary tuberculosis may also be seen in patients with malignant neoplasms or in those receiving chemotherapy for their malignancies.[6]

Atypical mycobacteria cause the vast majority of mycobacterial skin infections in immunosuppressed hosts. Skin lesions occur in more than 10% of all cases of disseminated atypical mycobacterial disease, and skin disease is the sole manifestation of mycobacterial disease in 12% of patients.[3] Since many atypical mycobacteria are environmental organisms, extremity lesions are most common. As opposed to the immunocompetent patient, however, from whom a history of trauma at the initial

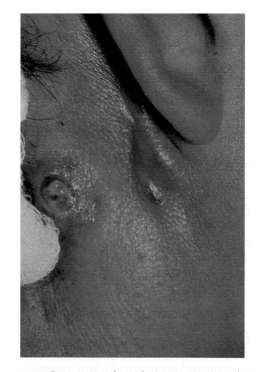

Figure 17.5 Cutaneous tuberculosis. A patient with Hodgkin's disease developed dermal and subcutaneous nodules. (Courtesy of Dr. Rocio Orozco-Topete.)

Aspergillosis

Aspergillosis, the second most common opportunistic fungal infection in immunocompromised hosts, can present in the skin as a primary cutaneous infection or as a consequence of dissemination from a visceral source, usually the lung. Most disseminated cases are due to *Aspergillus fumigatus*, but *Aspergillus flavus* causes most cases of primary cutaneous disease. Neutropenia, as with candidiasis, is the major risk factor, but immunosuppression and administration of broad-spectrum antibiotics also contribute.

Primary cutaneous aspergillosis frequently presents at a site of minor skin trauma occluded for some period by tape or a dressing. This is most typically an intravenous catheter site, especially an indwelling central venous catheter.[21] In some cases, the infecting organism can be cultured from the tape. Lesions present on the skin as grouped erythematous papules or papulopustules. They may be follicularly based. In leukemic children, lesions often occur on the palm and progress from papules to papulopustules to hemorrhagic bullae. If untreated, with persistent neutropenia, the lesions may progress to nodules. The diagnosis is confirmed by skin biopsy. A rapid bedside evaluation is potassium hydroxide examination of the roof of a bullous or pustular lesion, which will demonstrate the large septate branching hyphae. Treatment includes attempting to reverse the neutropenia, intravenous amphotericin B, and perhaps limited local excision of smaller lesions. Itraconazole, 400 mg daily, has been successful in some AIDS patients with single lesions we have managed. Primary cutaneous lesions can be the source of fatal visceral dissemination, so aggressive management is indicated.

Cutaneous lesions of disseminated aspergillosis are papules or subcutaneous nodules or abscesses. Lesions may develop necrosis centrally.[3] Diagnosis is by skin biopsy.

Fusarium *Infection*

Fusarium species have recently become an important fungal pathogen in immunocompromised hosts. Neutropenia is the major risk factor, followed by systemic corticosteroid therapy. *Fusarium* species may cause skin lesions from primary cutaneous inoculation or by dissemination. The toenails may be the source.[22] Localized disease may present as digital cellulitis adjacent to an infected toenail, papules, papulovesicles, crusts, ulcerations, or subcutaneous nodules. Disseminated disease presents with multiple, widespread lesions similar in morphology to those seen in primary disease. Necrosis of the center of the lesions is typical.[23,24] Diagnosis is by

skin biopsy. Treatment is with amphotericin B, but disseminated disease in the setting of immunosuppression is virtually always fatal.

VIRUSES

The cell-mediated immune system is critical in control of viral infections. The skin and mucosa are frequently parasitized by viruses in the setting of organ transplantation and HIV infection. Since certain viruses are oncogenic or important cofactors in oncogenesis, a complication of these viral infections can be mucocutaneous carcinomas.

HSV and molluscum contagiosum virus also affect persons with certain skin diseases, despite an apparent intact systemic cell-mediated immunity. Atopic dermatitis, Darier's disease, and benign familial pemphigus may all be complicated by widespread cutaneous herpes simplex (Kaposi's varicelliform eruption). Atopic dermatitis may also be complicated by molluscum contagiosum.

Herpes Simplex Virus

HSV types 1 and 2 are extremely prevalent infectious agents, which apparently remain in a latent state in all persons infected. In the setting of normal immunity, recurrences can be common but are usually of short duration with limited symptoms (see Ch. 15). In the setting of immunosuppression of the cell-mediated immune system by cytotoxic agents, corticosteroids, or congenital or acquired immunodeficiency, primary and recurrent disease is more severe, more persistent, and more symptomatic. In some settings (i.e., bone marrow transplantation), the risk of severe reactivation is so high that prophylactic systemic antivirals are administered. In the setting of immune suppression, any erosive mucocutaneous lesion should be considered herpes simplex until proved otherwise, especially lesions in the genital and orolabial regions. Atypical morphologies are also seen (Fig. 17.8).

Typically lesions appear as erosions or crusts. The early vesicular lesions may be transient or never seen. The three clinical hallmarks of herpes simplex infection are pain, an active vesicular border, and a scalloped periphery. Untreated erosive lesions may gradually expand (Fig. 17.9). In the oral mucosa, numerous erosions may be seen, involving all surfaces (as opposed to only the hard keratinized surfaces usually involved by recurrent oral herpes simplex). The tongue may be affected with geometric fissures on the central dorsal surface.[25] Rather than gradually expanding, mucocutaneous lesions may also appear and remain fixed and even become papular (Fig. 17.10). Herpetic whitlow, infection of the digit, presents as a painful paronychia that is initially vesicular and involves the lateral nail fold(s).[26] Untreated it may lead to loss of the nail and ulceration of a large portion of the digit.

Despite the frequent and severe skin infections caused by HSV in the immunosuppressed, visceral dissemination is unusual. Ocular involvement can occur from direct inoculation, and if lesions are present around the eye, careful ophthalmologic evaluation is required.

The diagnosis of herpes simplex is best confirmed by viral culture. Tzanck smear is rapid, but less sensitive, and does not distinguish HSV from varicella-zoster virus (VZV). Direct fluorescent antibody testing is specific and rapid. It is very useful in immunosuppressed hosts in whom therapeutic decisions need to be made expeditiously.

Therapy often can be instituted on clinical grounds pending confirmatory tests. Acyclovir is effective and safe. In patients with AIDS and those with persistent im-

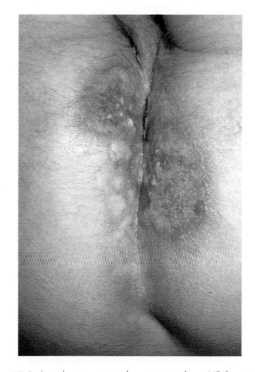

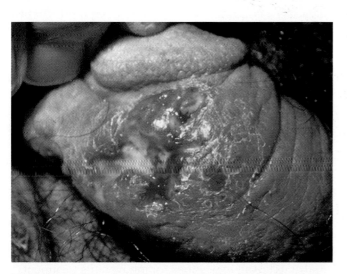

Figure 17.8 Herpes simplex. A leukemic patient with no prior history of genital herpes developed a nonhealing, purulent, deep ulceration. Cultures yielded only herpes simplex virus, and the lesion healed with oral acyclovir treatment.

Figure 17.9 Acyclovir-resistant herpes simplex. AIDS patient with expanding superficial ulceration perianally. Patient failed treatment with acyclovir, and the viral isolate lacked thymidine kinase.

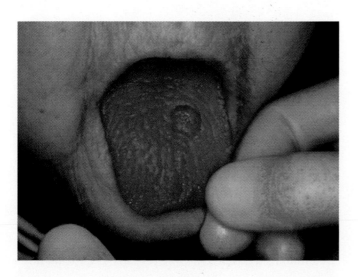

Figure 17.10 Herpes simplex. Papular lesion on the dorsum of the tongue in a patient with oat cell carcinoma.

munosuppression, consideration should be given to chronic suppressive therapy with acyclovir at a dosage of 400 mg bid.

Chronic treatment with acyclovir or treatment of large herpetic ulcerations may be complicated by the development of acyclovir resistance (see Fig. 17.9). The diagnosis is suspected when high doses of acyclovir do not rapidly lead to improvement. Viral isolates can be tested for acyclovir sensitivity. Treatment is with intravenous foscarnet.

Varicella-Zoster Virus

VZV causes primary infection (varicella, chickenpox) and recurrent disease (herpes zoster, shingles). Immunosuppression of the cell-mediated immune system leads to more frequent and more severe expression of primary and recurrent disease.

Varicella can be extremely severe and even fatal in the immunosuppressed. Varicella may be complicated by pneumonia, hepatitis, and encephalitis. Prior varicella does not always protect the immunosuppressed host from recurrent outbreaks.[27] The skin lesions in the immunosuppressed host are usually identical to varicella in the healthy host, beginning as 1 to 3-mm papules, which over 24 hours develop a small blister on an erythematous base. The number of lesions may be numerous in the immunosuppressed (Fig. 17.11). In the setting of immunosuppression, however, the lesions more frequently become necrotic, and ulceration may occur. Even if the lesions are few, the size of the lesion may be large (up to several centimeters), and necrosis of the full thickness of dermis may occur.

The diagnosis of varicella is by Tzanck smear or direct fluorescent antibody (DFA) testing. VZV grows slowly, and viral culture is often too slow to be useful clinically, making DFA extremely useful in establishing the diagnosis.

Ideally, treatment of varicella would involve prevention through the use of varicella vaccination if possible prior to immunosuppression. Intravenous acyclovir at a dosage of 10 mg/kg tid is given as soon as the diagnosis is suspected. Varicella-zoster immune globulin may be given if the patient has severe life-threatening disease and is not responding to acyclovir.

Herpes zoster occurs much more commonly in the immunosuppressed host.[28–30] In HIV-infected men, the risk for developing zoster is increased 25-fold and in cancer patients about 5-fold. The clinical appearance is usually identical to typical zoster, but the lesions may be more ulcerative and necrotic and may scar more

severely (Fig. 17.12). In AIDS patients, ocular and neurologic complications of herpes zoster are increased. Immunosuppressed patients often have recurrences of zoster, up to 25% in patients with AIDS. Visceral dissemination and fatal outcome are extremely rare in immunosuppressed patients (about 0.3%), but cutaneous dissemination is not uncommon, occurring in 12% of cancer patients, especially those with hematologic malignancies.

Two atypical patterns of zoster have been described in AIDS patients: (1) ecthymatous lesions punched out ulcerations with a central crust, and (2) verrucous lesions (Fig. 17.13). These patterns were not reported prior to the AIDS epidemic. These atypical clinical patterns, especially the verrucous pattern, may correlate with acyclovir resistance.

The diagnosis of dermatomal zoster can be made clinically and confirmed by DFA if required. Atypical and disseminated cases need to be confirmed to rule out disseminated HSV. Therapy should be begun on suspicion and the appropriate tests sent as confirmation.

In the immunosuppressed host, all cases of herpes zoster should be treated with an antiviral, even if treatment is started more than 96 hours after onset. Oral acyclovir at a dosage of 800 mg five times daily is the most carefully studied. Famciclovir at a dosage of 500 mg tid or valacyclovir 1 gm tid can also be used. Systemic corticosteroids should probably be avoided in the immunosuppressed, even with painful zoster, since they may increase the risk of dissemination.

In certain settings, intravenous acyclovir should be given. Involvement of the V1 trigeminal dermatome, ocular involvement, Ramsay Hunt syndrome, and failure of antivirals are all indications for intravenous treatment. In chronic lesions not responding to intravenous acyclovir, the possibility of acyclovir resistance should be entertained. Treatment is with intravenous foscarnet.

Cytomegalovirus

Cytomegalovirus (CMV) infection in the skin is uncommon. Clinically CMV usually is described as causing superficial ulcerations or fissures of the oral or anal area in the immunosuppressed host.[31] Erosive diaper dermatitis is also described in the setting of HIV disease. The lesions are clinically identical to HSV or VZV skin lesions or appear like aphthous ulceration. Concurrent CMV viremia has been variably present, and CMV retinitis often is not found. When anal ulceration occurs, CMV colitis may or may not coexist. The diagnosis is usually established by histologically identifying specific "cytopathic CMV" effect in blood vessels in a skin lesion. Determining a pathogenic role for CMV is difficult, how-

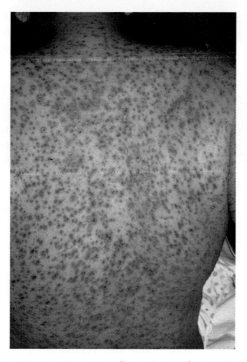

Figure 17.11 Varicella. Patient with stage IV Hodgkin's disease. Patient developed thousands of necrotic skin lesions as well as varicella pneumonia.

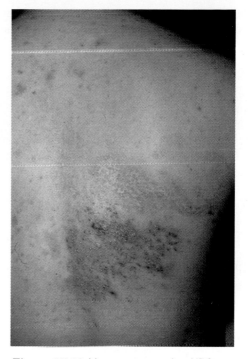

Figure 17.12 Herpes zoster. An AIDS patient with a painful, dermatomal eruption. Note the dermatomal scar above the vesicular eruption representing scarring from a previous episode of herpes zoster.

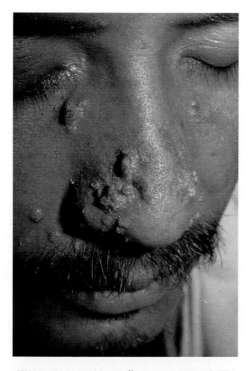

Figure 17.13 Varicella zoster virus (VZV). Widespread verrucous papules, which histologically showed "herpes virus" changes in epidermis. Cultures isolated acyclovir-resistant VZV.

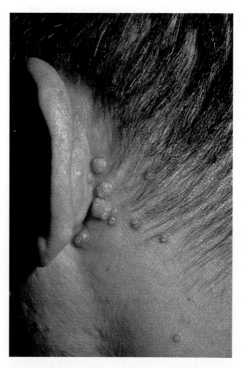

Figure 17.14 Molluscum contagiosum. AIDS patient with asymptomatic pearly papules with central umbilication on the head and neck.

ever, since CMV may be expressed in inflamed skin without being the primary pathogen. Polymerase chain reaction and DNA hybridization may identify CMV in the tissue but do not prove its pathogenicity. Specific treatment for the CMV with ganciclovir or foscarnet may not lead to improvement. Such therapies are also effective against HSV and VZV, making it difficult to conclude that eradication of CMV led to improvement of the ulcerative lesion. Until this situation is further defined, the diagnosis of CMV ulceration should not be made until all other diagnostic possibilities have been excluded. Such ulcerations should be managed with antiherpetic agents: initially high doses of acyclovir (doses effective for VZV) and if this fails, foscarnet. Lesions failing antiviral therapy may be considered aphthous equivalents and treated with topical or intralesional corticosteroids.

Other described patterns include cutaneous purpura (either palpable or nonpalpable) and one case of a purpuric vesiculobullous eruption. In the latter case, CMV was reported to have been cultured from the skin, but the isolated virus was not identified by specific antisera.

Molluscum Contagiosum Virus

This poxvirus is a common cutaneous pathogen in the setting of AIDS but is uncommon in other forms of immunosuppression. Molluscum contagiosum tends to appear when the T-helper cell count is below 200 mm³, and the severity of infection tends to parallel the stage of HIV disease. Most patients with extensive molluscum or molluscum in more than one anatomic site have T-helper cell counts below 50.[32]

Various clinical patterns of molluscum contagiosum have been describe in HIV (Fig. 17.14). Lesions may be larger than those seen in the healthy host, measuring larger than 1 cm and resembling a basal cell carcinoma or even a keratoacanthoma. Coalescent lesions may form tumors that distort facial features. Lesions may also be smaller, appearing as sheets of tiny papules less than 1 mm in size. On close inspection, lesions are noted to be follicular. Lesions involve the face and genitalia primarily, with scattered lesions on the trunk. On the face and neck, the beard area and the periorbital area are often primarily involved. In the genitalia, the penis, scrotum, perianal area, and proximal thighs are affected. Extension onto the oral or genital mucosa is uncommon and almost diagnostic of a T-helper cell count less than 50.

Treatment is destructive; no specific antivirals are available for molluscum contagiosum. Results of treatment are dependent on the health and immune status of the host. Cryotherapy, cantharidin, electrocautery, topical 5-fluorouracil, and trichloroacetic acid peels have all been used.

The application of 13-*cis* retinoic acid nightly at the highest concentration tolerated appears to slow down the rate of appearance of new lesions in some patients.

REFERENCES

1. El Baze P, Thyss A, Vinti H et al: A study of nineteen immunocopromised patients with extensive skin lesions caused by *Pseudomonas aeruginosa* with and without bacteremia. Acta Derm Venereol 71:411, 1991

2. Fergie JE, Patrick CC, Lott L: *Pseudomonas aeruginosa* cellulitis and ecthyma gangrenosum in immunocompromised children. Pediatr Dis J 10:496, 1991

3. Gentry LO, Zeluff B, Kielhofner, MA: Dermatologic manifestations of infectious diseases in cardiac patients. Infect Dis Clin North Am 8:637, 1994

4. Arduino RC, Johnson PC, Miranda AG: Nocardiosis in rena transplant recipients undergoing immunosuppression with cyclosporine. Clin Infect Dis 16:505, 1993

5. Stack RJ, Bickley LK, Coppel IG: Military tuberculosis presenting as skin lesions in a patient with acquired immunodeficiency syndrome. J Am Acad Dermatol 23:103, 1990

6. Asnis DS, Bresciani AR: Cutaneous tuberculosis: a rare presentation of malignancy. Clin Infect Dis 15:158, 1992

7. Enzenauer RJ, McKoy J, Vincent D, Gates R: Disseminated cutaneous and synovial. *Mycobacterium marinum* infection is a patient with systemic lupus erythematosus. South Med J 83:471, 1990

8. Patel R, Roberts GD, Keating MR, Paya CV: Infections due to nontuberculous mycobacteria in kidney, heart, and liver transplant recipients. Clin Infect Dis 19:263, 1994

9. Stellbrink HJ, Koperski K, Albrecht H, Greten H: *Mycobacterium kansasii* infection limited to skin and lymph node in a patient with AIDS. Clin Exp Dermatol 15:457, 1990

10. Breathnach A, Level N, Munro C, Natarajan S, Pedler S: Cutaneous *Mycobacterium kansasii* infection: case report and review. Clin Infect Dis 20:812, 1995

11. Brandwein M, Choi HS, Strauchen J, Stoler M, Jagirdar J: Spindle cell reaction to nontuberculosis mycobacteriosis in AIDs mimicking a spindle cell neoplasm. Virchows Arch A Pathol Anat Histopathol 416:281, 1990

12. Jacobson MA: Disseminated *Mycobacterium avium* complex and other bacterial infections. In Sande

MA, Volderding PA (eds): The Medical Management of AIDS. 4th Ed. WB Saunders, Philadelphia, 1995

13. Williams JT, Pulitzer DR, DeVillez RL: Papulonecrotic tuberculid secondary to disseminated *Mycobacterium avium* complex Int J Dermatol 33:109, 1994

14. Barbaro DJ, Orcutt VL, Coldiron BM: *Mycobacterium avium-Mycobacterium intracellulare* infection limited to the skin and lymph nodes in patients with AIDS. Rev Infect Dis 11:625, 1989

15. Wallace RJ, Brown BA, Onyi GO: Skin, soft tissue, and bone infections due to *Mycobacterium chelone-ichelonei*: importance of prior corticosteroid therapy, frequency of disseminated infections, and resistance to oral antimicrobials other than clarithromycin. J Infect Dis 166:405, 1992

16. Singh N, Rihs JD, Gayowski T, Yu VL: Cutaneous crystococcosis mimicking bacterial cellulitis in a liver transplant recipient: case report and review in solid organ transplant recipients. Clin Transplant 8:365, 1994

17. Murakawa GJ, McCalmont T, Altman J et al: Disseminated acanthamebiasis in patients with AIDS: a report of five cases and a review of the literature. Arch Dermatol 131:1291, 1995

18. Wheat J, Connolly-Stringfield PA, Baker RL et al: Disseminated histoplasmosis in AIDS: clinical findings, diagnosis and treatment, and review of the literature. Medicine (Baltimore) 69:361, 1993

19. Johnson PC, Khardori N, Najjar AF et al: Progressive disseminated histoplasmosis in patients with AIDS. Am J Med 85:152, 1988

20. Wheat J, Hafner R, Wulfsohn M et al: Prevention of relapse of histoplasmosis with traconazole in patients with the acquired immunodeficiency syndrome. Ann Intern Med 118:610, 1993

21. Hunt SJ, Nagi C, Gross KG, Wong DS, Mathews WC: Primary cutaneous aspergillosis near central venous catheters in patients with AIDS. Arch Dermatol 128:1229, 1992

22. Girmenia C, Arcese W, Micozzi A et al: Onychomycosis as a possible origin of disseminated *Fusarium solani* infection in a patient with severe aplastic anemia. Clin Infect Dis 14:1167, 1992

23. Merz WG, Karp JE, Hoagland M et al: Diagnosis and successful treatment of fusariosis in the compromised host. J Infect Dis 158:1046, 1988

24. Nelson PE, Dignani MC, Anaissie EJ: Taxonomy, biology, and clinical aspects of *Fusarium* species. Clin Microbiol Rev 7:479, 1994

25. Grossman ME, Stevens AW, Cohen PR: Brief report: Herpetic geometric glossitis N Engl J Med 329:1859, 1993

26. Zuretti AR, Schwartz IS: Gangrenous herpetic whitlow in a HIV-positive patient. Am J Clin Pathol 93:828, 1990

27. Baxter JD, DiNubile MJ: Relapsing chickenpox in a young man with non-Hodgkin's lymphoma. Clin Infect Dis 18:785, 1994

28. Rusthoven JJ, Ahlgren P, Elhakim T et al: Varicella-zoster infection in adult cancer patients: a population study Arch Intern Med 148:1561, 1988

29. Glesby MJ, Moore RD, Chaisson RE: Clinical spectrum of herpes zoster in adults infected with HIV. Clin Infect Dis 21:370, 1995

30. Buchbinder SP, Katz MH, Hessol NA et al: Herpes zoster and HIV infection. J Infect Dis 166:1153, 1992

31. Puy-Montbrun T, Ganansia R, Lemarchand N, Delechenault P, Denis J: Anal ulcerations due to cytomegalovirus in patients with AIDS: report of six cases. Dis Colon Rectum 33:1041, 1990

32. Schwartz JJ, Myskowski PL: Molluscum contagiosum in patients with HIV infection: a review of twenty-seven patients. J Am Acad Dermatol 27:583, 1992

SUGGESTED READING

Grossman ME, Roth J: Cutaneous Manifestations of Infection in the Immunocompromised Host. Williams & Wilkins, Baltimore, 1995

Radents WH: Continuing medical education: opportunistic fungal infections in immunocompromised hosts. J Am Acad Dermatol 20:989, 1989

CHAPTER 18

Human Papillomavirus Infection

Mary M. Christian

Tanya Y. Evans

Stephen K. Tyring

SUMMARY

Etiology Over 70 types of human papillomavirus (HPV)

Clinical Features Cutaneous warts (common, flat, plantar, filiform, and anogenital warts; bowenoid papulosis); extracutaneous warts (oral, laryngeal, and cervical warts); epidermodysplasia verruciformis (flat wart-like lesions, pityriasis versicolor–like lesions, seborrheic keratotic–like lesions, skin cancers)

Pathology Hyperkeratosis, parakeratosis, papillomatosis, acanthosis, and koilocytotic atypia, thrombosed dermal capillaries

Diagnosis Clinical, histopathologic, and molecular methods.

Treatment Destruction (cryotherapy, carbon-dioxide laser, acid preparations, podophyllin, podophyllotoxin, bleomycin), surgery (excision, electrocautery, electrodesiccation, curettage), and antiviral/immunomodulatory drugs (interferons, retinoids, cimetidine, Imiquimod, cidofovir).

Differential Diagnosis Common warts (seborrheic keratoses, actinic keratoses, squamous cell carcinoma); extensive verruca (arsenical keratoses and punctate keratoderma); flat warts (lichen nitidus, lichen planus, lichen striatus, syringomas, acrokeratosis verruciformis); plantar warts (acquired digital fibrokeratomas, clavi, foreign body reactions); condylomata accuminata (condylomata lata); bowenoid papulosis (seborrheic keratoses, melanocytic nevi)

ETIOLOGY

There are over 70 types of human papillomavirus (HPV) (Table 18.1). The papillomaviruses are double-stranded DNA viruses of the Papovaviridae family. Other members of this family include polyomavirus, BK virus, and JC virus. The papillomavirus carries supercoiled, circular DNA within an icosahedral capsid. Because the capsid is not surrounded by an envelope, the virus is resistant to desiccation, freezing, and ether inactivation.[1] Papillomaviruses are highly host specific and do not produce disease in heterologous species. The infection site and disease course are determined by the HPV type. While most HPVs cause self-limited hyperproliferative lesions (known as warts), others are precursors of malignancy. HPVs associated with a high risk of malignancy include types 5, 8, 16, 18, 30, 31, 33, 35, 39, 45, 51, 52, 55, 56, 58, and 68; those associated with a low risk include types 6, 11, 34, 40, 42–44, 53, 54, 57, and 59.[2,3]

CLINICAL FEATURES

Cutaneous

Common warts (verruca vulgaris) are firm, rough, keratotic papules that may develop on any skin surface. The dorsum of the hands and fingers are the most common

---

CLINICAL TYPES OF HPV

Cutaneous
   Common warts
   Flat warts
   Plantar warts
   Filiform warts
   Anogenital warts
   Bowenoid papulosis

Extracutaneous
   Oral warts
   Laryngeal warts
   Cervical warts

Epidermodysplasia Verruciformis
   Flat lesions
   Pityriasis versicolor–like lesions
   Seborrheic keratotic–like lesions
   Skin cancers

Table 18.1 HPV Types and Clinical Associations

HPV-1	Plantar warts; common warts	HPV-26–29	Flat warts; common warts
HPV-2	Common warts; flat warts	HPV-30	Laryngeal carcinoma; anogenital warts
HPV-3	Flat warts; epidermodysplasia verruciformis (EV)	HPV-31–32	Anogenital warts; cervical dysplasia and carcinoma; bowenoid papulosis, focal epithelial hyperplasia
HPV-4	Common warts; plantar warts	HPV-33	Cervical carcinoma; genital intraepithelial neoplasia
HPV-5	EV		
HPV-6	Anogenital warts; laryngeal warts; verrucous carcinoma	HPV-34	Bowen's disease; bowenoid papulosis
HPV-7	Meat handler's hand warts	HPV-35	Cervical dysplasia and carcinoma
HPV-8	EV	HPV-36	EV
HPV-9	EV; keratocanthomas	HPV-37	Keratocanthomas; EV
HPV-10	Flat warts; EV	HPV-38	EV
HPV-11	Anogenital warts; laryngeal warts; verrucous carcinoma	HPV-39	Bowenoid papulosis; cervical carcinoma
		HPV-41	Flat warts
HPV-12	EV	HPV-42	Anogenital warts; cervical dysplasia and carcinoma; bowenoid papulosis
HPV-13	Oral focal epithelial hyperplasia		
HPV-14	EV	HPV-43–44	Anogenital warts; laryngeal warts
HPV-15	EV	HPV-46–47	EV
HPV-16	Anogenital warts; cervical dysplasia and carcinoma: bowenoid papulosis	HPV-48	Bowen's disease; bowenoid papulosis
		HPV-49–50	EV
HPV-17	EV	HPV-51–54	Anogenital warts; cervical dysplasia and carcinoma; bowenoid papulosis
HPV-18	Anogenital warts; cervical dysplasia and carcinoma; bowenoid papulosis	HPV-55	Anogenital warts; laryngeal warts
HPV-19–25	EV		

(Data from Cobb[1]; Miller[6]; and Howley PM, Schlegel R: The human papillomavirus. Am J Med 85:155, 1988.)

sites (Fig. 18.1), except in children under 12, where the knees are the favored area.[1] Isolated or grouped lesions may occur. While most warts are asymptomatic, the size and location may complicate the course. Periungal and subungal warts may interfere with nail plate growth and be recalcitrant to therapy.

Flat warts (verruca plana) are smooth, slightly raised papules that typically develop on the face, dorsal hands, and shins (Fig. 18.2). They are flesh-colored, gray, red, or brown in color. One to several hundreds of lesions may occur. Because of a predilection for Koebner's phenomenon, linear arrangements are common.[1,4]

Plantar warts are rough keratotic papules that develop on the soles of the feet. Because they often form below pressure points, pain may be associated. Coalescing warts are termed a mosaic wart (Fig. 18.3), whereas an endophytic, deep wart is called a myrimecia.[1,4]

Filiform warts are flesh-colored, slender papules with "fingerlike" projections that extend from a narrow base (Fig. 18.4). Development around the mouth, ala nasi, and eyes is common.

Anogenital warts are typically soft, pink, cauliflower-like lesions (Figs. 18.5 and 18.6). The term *condyloma accuminatum* (which means "pointed knuckle") is often used (Fig. 18.7). Sessile or keratotic papules may also occur (Fig. 18.8). The sites of predilection in men are the glans (Fig. 18.9), corona, and frenulum, and in women, the posterior introitus.[4]

Bowenoid papulosis manifests as multiple 2- to 3-mm, velvety, pigmented papules that develop on the skin or mucous membranes of the anogenital area. Young adults are affected most frequently, though any age group may be affected. There is often a history of anogenital warts.[4] Because the lesions may harbor HPV-16 (an oncogenic strain), aggressive therapy is recommended.[5]

Figure 18.1 Common warts on the dorsal hands and fingers of a child.

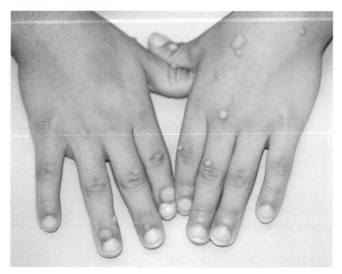

Figure 18.2 Flat warts on the shin.

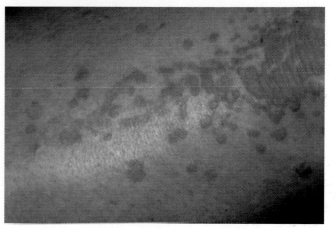

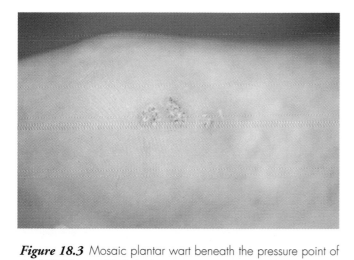

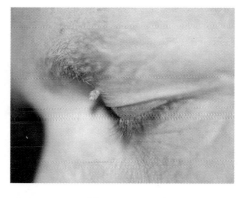

Figure 18.4 Filliform wart on the upper eyelid.

Figure 18.3 Mosaic plantar wart beneath the pressure point of the first metatarsal head.

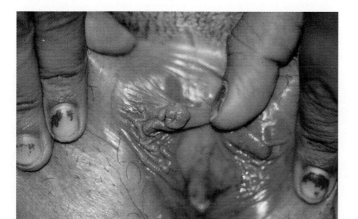

Figure 18.5 Pedunculated cauliflower-like wart on the right labia minora.

Figure 18.6 Cauliflower-like warts on the medial thighs. This patient also had extensive perianal and penile warts.

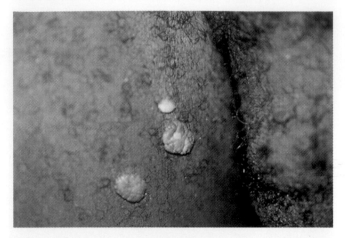

Figure 18.7 Perianal condylomata accuminata resembling "pointed knuckles."

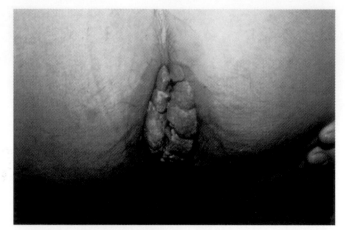

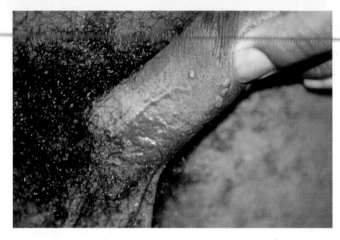

Figure 18.8 Sessile papular warts on the penile shaft.

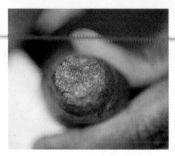

Figure 18.9 Verrucous ring of warts encircling the glans. Circumcision was required to correct the phimosis that developed after the growth of these lesions.

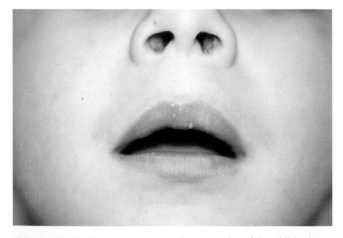

Figure 18.10 Common warts on the upper lip of the child whose hands are shown in Figure 18.1. Thumb sucking was the suspected route of transmission.

Extracutaneous (Mucosal)

Verruca vulgaris and condyloma accuminatum may develop in the mouth. Clinically, they resemble their cutaneous counterparts.[6] Oral verruca vulgaris typically occurs in children with hand warts who self-inoculate themselves (Fig. 18.10). Oral condyloma accuminatum is transmitted through sexual contact or self-inoculation. Oral focal epithelial hyperplasia, or Heck's disease, was first described in Native American children. Since then, cases in other races have been reported, and it is common in whites. Multiple white or mucosal-colored soft papules develop on the buccal, gingival, or labial mucosa.[1] In oral florid papillomatosis, white cauliflower-like lesions characteristically develop in the oral cavity of elderly patients. This entity is strongly associated with verrucous carcinoma.

Laryngeal (respiratory) papillomatosis is an uncommon but potential life-threatening entity. It occurs in children and adults, but rarely in adolescents. Hoarseness and stridor are common presenting signs. The papillomas typically involve the larynx. Extension into the oropharyngeal or bronchopulmonary tracts may occur. Enlargement of the lesions may result in airway obstruction and death.[1] Cervical warts are flat lesions that may require colposcopy for visualization. The gradual progression of cervical warts to cervical dysplasia, carcinoma in situ, and cervical carcinoma is strongly supported.

Epidermodysplasia Verruciformis

Epidermodysplasia verruciformis (EV) is a rare disease characterized by refractory, persistent HPV infection. It typically begins during childhood. The inheritance pattern is usually autosomal recessive. While the disease mechanism is unknown, a defect in a tumor suppressor gene has been proposed.[7] The cutaneous manifestations include flat wart–like lesions, pityriasis versicolor–like lesions, seborrheic keratosis–like lesions, and skin cancers. Seborrheic keratosis–like lesions develop on sun-exposed skin and may be precancerous.[8] Bowen's disease and squamous cell carcinomas develop in approximately 30% of EV patients after 25 years of disease.[9] They occur almost exclusively in sun-exposed areas, suggesting that ultraviolet radiation is a cocarcinogen with the EV HPVs.[1]

PATHOLOGY

In common warts, hyperkeratosis, acanthosis, and papillomatosis are present. Tiers of parakeratosis over the papillomatous epidermal elevations and aggregates of keratohyaline granules in the epidermal valleys are evident.[1] HPV-infected keratinocytes in the stratum spinosum and stratum granulosum are vacuolated, with basophilic nuclei, perinuclear halos, and pale cytoplasm. These vacuolated cells are termed koilocytes and are characteristic of HPV-infected cells (Fig. 18.11). Flat warts lack significant papillomatosis and parakeratosis (Fig. 18.12). In myrimecial plantar warts, cytoplasmic eosinophilic keratohyaline granules are present (Fig. 18.13). Anogenital warts display pseudoepitheliomatous hyperplasia and more pronounced acanthosis than common warts.[1] Bowenoid papulosis resembles Bowen's disease histologically, with a "windblown" epidermis and dyskeratotic keratinocytes.[10] Oral florid papillomatosis shows upward verrucous projections and downward club-shaped extensions of the epithelium.[10]

DIAGNOSIS

Most cutaneous HPV infections can be diagnosed by clinical appearance. The loss of skin surface lines and the presence of punctate black dots are characteristic features (Fig. 18.14). The black dots reflect thrombosed capillaries in the dermal papillae and may become more evident with paring. Deep paring will reveal foci of bleeding (Fig. 18.15). The application of 5% acetic acid gives warts an "acetowhite" appearance (Fig. 18.16). This may be helpful in diagnosing subtle lesions, though it is not specific for HPV disease.[3]

Molecular methods have been developed for identifying and typing HPV DNA. Techniques utilized include true in situ hybridization, hybrid capture, Southern blot, and dot blot assays.[3] The polymerase chain reaction (PCR) amplifies DNA, so that a single DNA molecule can be detected in as many as 10^5 cells.[1] PCR significantly increases the sensitivity of testing. However, because DNA contaminants can also be amplified, the false-positive rate increases when this method is utilized. The risk of contamination with extraneous DNA can be minimized by meticulous specimen collection, careful processing, and negative controls.[3]

TREATMENT

Numerous modalities exist for the treatment of warts (Table 18.2). While every wart does not need to be treated, some should be aggressively eradicated because of the oncogenicity of certain HPVs. The modality chosen by the patient and physician is dependent on the age of the patient, the location of the wart, the extent of disease, and the suspected HPV type. Pain, risk of scar-

Figure 18.11 Verruca vulgaris. Hyperkeratosis, parakeratosis, acnathosis, papillomatosis, and koilocytic change are present in the epidermis.

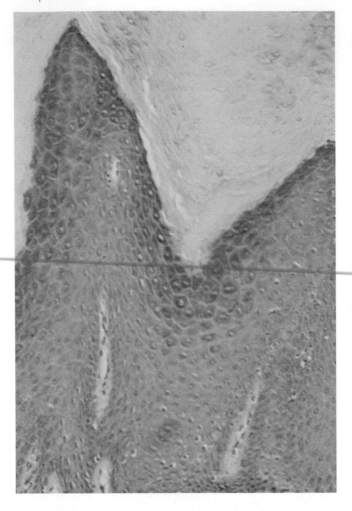

Figure 18.13 Myrimecial plantar wart. Eosinophilic cytoplasmic keratohyaline granules are characteristic.

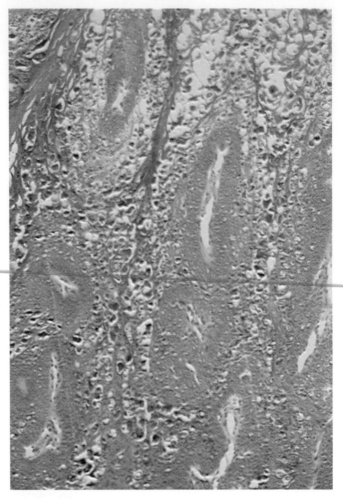

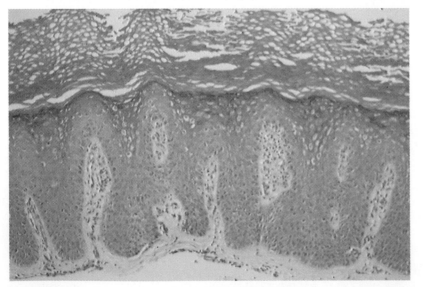

Figure 18.12 Verruca plana. Koilocytic change is evident in the upper stratum malpighii; papillomatosis and parakeratosis are minimal.

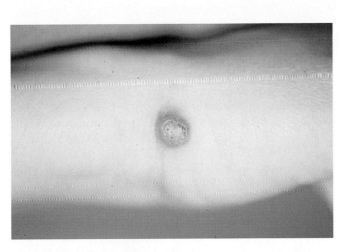

Figure 18.14 Punctate black dots and loss of skin surface lines are evident in this wart.

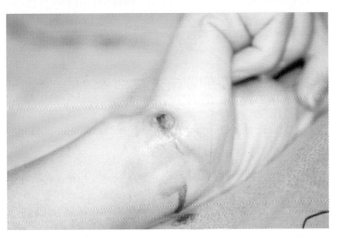

Figure 18.15 Foci of bleeding were evident after shaving the wart shown in Figure 18.14.

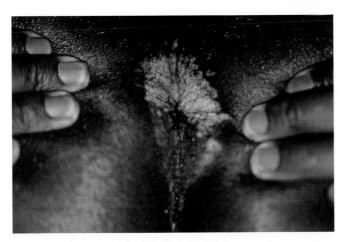

Figure 18.16 These perianal warts became "acetowhite" after applying 5% acetic acid.

Table 18.2 Summary of Treatment for HPV Warts

Destruction by cryotherapy, carbon-dioxide laser, acids, podophyllin, podophyllotoxin, bleomycin

Excision, electrocautery, electrodesiccation, and curettage surgical techniques

Antiviral/immunomodulatory drugs such as interferons, retinoids, cimetidine, imiquimod, and cidofovir

ring, likelihood of recurrence, and cost are also factors to be considered.

Destruction through cryotherapy is a mainstay of therapy for warts. Local tissue destruction and immune system stimulation are the presumed mechanisms of action.[11] The lesion and a 2- to 3-mm rim of normal tissue should be frozen. Warts become white during treatment and retain this appearance longer than the surrounding skin (Fig. 18.17). The "thaw time" of the lesion should not exceed 30 seconds. Several minutes after treatment, a halo of mild erythema develops (Fig. 18.18). This indicates adequate treatment and appropriate technique. Side effects include pain, necrosis, blistering, ulceration, and postinflammatory hyper- or hypopigmentation.[11] Scarring is uncommon in warts frozen for less than 30 seconds, though it can occur (Fig. 18.19). Reports of damage to underlying structures (such as nerves on the sides of fingers) have been made.[4] The carbon-dioxide laser is useful for treating refractory cases and offers the advantage of fine control of the depth and width of destruction (Fig. 18.20). Chemical destruction using cantharidin (an extract from the green blister beetle) or an acid preparation (such as lactic acid, trichloroacetic acid, salicyclic acid, or retinoic acid) is an economic and sometimes effective approach.

Podophyllin was a common therapy for condylomata acuminata. It is derived from the roots of the plant *Podophyllum peltatum*. It may be self-administered but usually is not due to the risk of neurotoxicity. Because of the adverse reactions (both local and systemic) and the variable success rates reported with podophyllin, its use is limited. Podofilox, the active ingredient in podophyllin, was approved in 1991 by the Food and Drug Administration for the treatment of condylomata acuminata. It is more effective than podophyllin (94% effective compared with 29%) and carries a lower recurrence rate (23% versus 38%). In addition, it is locally less irritating than podophyllin and not associated with any adverse systemic reactions.

Bleomycin is an antiproliferative agent that may be used for severe, recalcitrant warts. Local anesthesia is required for intralesional therapy. The wart blanches with injection, and a hemorrhagic eschar subsequently develops. Cure rates of 75% have been reported with bleomycin in previously refractory lesions. Onychodystrophy, nail loss, and Raynaud's phenomenon have been reported following treatment of nail and finger lesions.

Surgical removal or destruction of warts is very effective, though usually a last resort due to the pain, increased cost, and scarring that occur. In general, patients treated with excision, electrocautery, electrodesiccation, or curettage have fewer recurrences and need fewer treatments than those treated with cryotherapy (Fig. 18.21). Surgical excision of first-occurrence condylomata acuminata was superior to podophyllin in one study, with fewer recurrences occurring in the surgically treated group (29% compared to 65%) at 12 months.[11]

Interferons-α, β, and γ have been used alone and in combination with other modalities to treat anogenital warts. The efficacy achieved with interferon (IFN) is dependent on the infecting HPV type and the patient's ability to mount an immune response. Low response rates occur in patients with extensive lesions due to HPV-16 or HPV-18 and in patients with human immunodeficiency virus (HIV) infection. In contrast, high response rates have been achieved with IFN monotherapy in small warts caused by HPV-6 or HPV-11 that were present for less than 3 months.[12] While the ideal regimen, dosage, and duration of IFN is not established for the treatment of anogenital warts, a complete response in 40 to 60% of patients receiving between 1 and 5 million units of IFN-α or IFN-β three times per week for 4 to 8 weeks has been reported.[12] Although IFN is not cost-effective in all cases, it is efficacious in immunocompetent patients with refractory or extensive anogenital warts.

Retinoids are being used to treat HPV in immunocompromised patients. In a patient with sarcoidosis and extensive warts associated with corticosteroid therapy, etretinate, 100 mg/day, resulted in a dramatic resolution of the warts; tapering below 30 mg/day led to a recurrence. In a patient with EV, Lutzner[13] described a decrease in several tumors' sizes and a resolution of most of the patient's flat wart–like lesions. Enhancement of humoral and cell-mediated immunity and regulation of cellular differentiation are proposed mechanisms of action.[1]

Imiquimod is an immune enhancing drug that stimulates the production of IFN-α and other cytokines. A 56% anogenital wart clearance rate has been reported with the application of 5% cream 3 days a week for up

Figure 18.17 Cryotherapy of recurrent warts at a previously treated site.

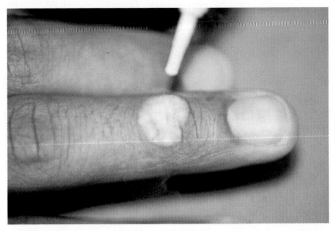

Figure 18.18 Mild perilesional erythema following cryotherapy.

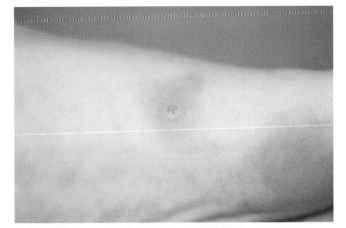

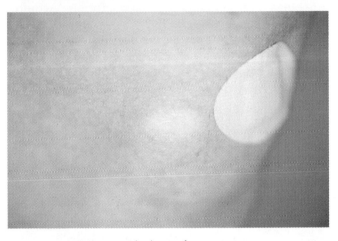

Figure 18.19 A scar on the knee of a young woman many years after aggressive cryotherapy of a wart during childhood.

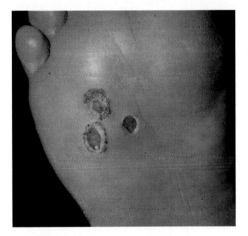

Figure 18.20 Post carbon-dioxide laser treatment of multiple plantar warts.

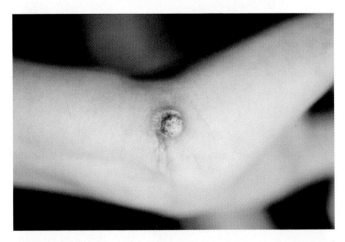

Figure 18.21 Appearance of the wart shown in Figure 18.14 after electrodesiccation and curettage.

to 16 weeks.[14] Imiquimod cream 5% is more effective than lower concentrations, though local skin reactions (typically erythema) are more common.[15] Other therapies for HPV infections are being studied. Cimetidine is an H_2 receptor antagonist that presumably enhances cell-mediated immunity by blocking H_2 receptors on T-suppressor cells. Reports of recalcitrant common warts in children and adults resolving with high-dose cimetidine have been made[16] (Figs. 18.22 and 18.23). A recent double-blind, placebo-controlled study in Turkey with 70 patients reported no significant difference between the cimetidine and placebo groups.[17] More studies are needed to determine the true efficacy of cimetidine.

During a 12 week follow-up period the recurrence rate in patients who experienced total clearance with 5% imiquimod cream was only 13%, a figure that is considered low compared to other forms of therapy. Cidofovir (previously known as HPMPC) is a nucleotide analog with potent antiviral activity against the herpesviruses, papillomaviruses, and other DNA viruses. Phase II and III studies revealed that intravenous cidofovir slowed the progression of previously untreated and relapsing cytomegalovirus retinitis in acquired immunodeficiency syndrome (AIDS) patients. Topical cidofovir is currently being evaluated for the treatment of herpes genitalis and anogenital HPV infections in AIDS patients.[18] Preliminary results appear promising. Development of a subunit vaccine for genital HPV infection is under way. The viral E6 and E7 oncoproteins and the L1 major capsid protein are the possible targets.[19]

DIFFERENTIAL DIAGNOSIS

Common warts must be distinguished from seborrheic keratoses (Fig. 18.24), actinic keratoses (Fig. 18.25), and squamous cell carcinomas. Extensive verruca may resemble arsenical keratoses and punctate keratoderma (Fig. 18.26). The differential diagnosis of flat warts includes lichen nitidus, lichen planus, lichen striatus, syringomas, and acrokeratosis verruciformis. Acquired digital fibrokeratomas (Fig. 18.27), clavi (Fig. 18.28), and foreign body reactions may resemble plantar warts. Condylomata accuminata should not be confused with the moist, smooth papules of condylomata lata. Bowenoid papulosis may resemble seborrheic keratoses and melanocytic nevi.

Figure 18.22 Recalcitrant wart on a woman's thumb before cimetidine treatment.

Figure 18.23 Resolution of wart shown in Figure 18.22 after high-dose cimetidine therapy for 6 weeks.

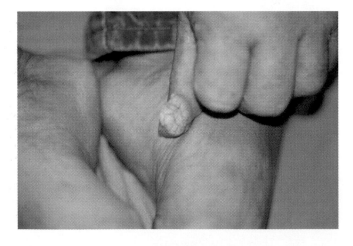

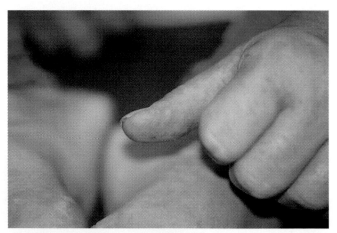

Figure 18.24 Seborrheic keratoses can be difficult to distinguish from warts, particularly when irritated (as this one was).

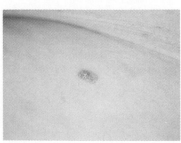

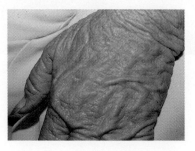

Figure 18.25 Actinic keratosis on the dorsal hand resembling a common wart. Both may be treated with cryotherapy.

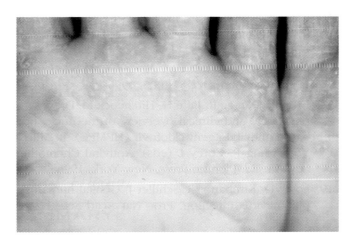

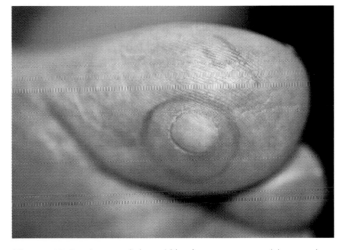

Figure 18.27 Acquired digital fibrokeratoma resembling a plantar wart.

Figure 18.26 Palmar punctate keratoderma.

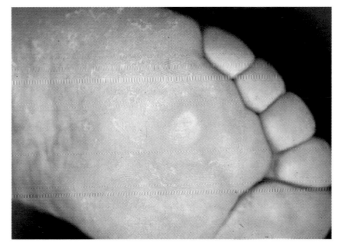

Figure 18.28 Corns may be difficult to distinguish from plantar warts. Paring to determine if black dots are present is a useful diagnostic tool.

REFERENCES

1. Cobb M: Human papillomavirus infection. J Am Acad Dermatol 22:547, 1990

2. McCance D: Human papillomaviruses. Infect Dis Clin North Am 8:751, 1994

3. Vittorio C, Schiffman M, Weinstock M: Epidemiology of human papillomaviruses. Dermatol Clin 13:561, 1995

4. Highet A, Kurtz J: Viral infections. In Champion R, Burton J, Ebling F (eds): Textbook of Dermatology. 5th Ed. Blackwell Scientific Publications, London, 1992

5. Lowy D, Androphy E: Warts. In Fitzpatrick T, Eisen A, Wolff K, Freedberg I, Austen K (eds): Dermatology in General Medicine. 4th Ed. McGraw-Hill, New York, 1993

6. Miller C: Herpes simplex virus and human papillomavirus infections of the oral cavity. Semin Dermatol 13:108, 1994

7. Jablonska S, Majewski S: Epidermodysplasia verruciformis: immunological and clinical aspects. Curr Top Microbiol Immunol 186:157, 1994

8. Tomasini C, Aloi F, Pippione M: Seborrheic keratosis–like lesions in epidermodysplasia verruciformis. J Cutan Pathol 20:237, 1993

9. Pfister H: Human papillomaviruses and skin cancer. Semin Cancer Biol 3:263, 1992

10. Lever WF, Schaumberg-Lever G: Histopathology of the Skin. 7th Ed. Lippincott, Philadelphia, 1990

11. Cowsert L: Treatment of papillomavirus infections: recent practice and future approaches. Intervirology 37:226, 1994

Table 19.1 Exanthems

DISEASE (ETIOLOGY)	USUAL AGE	SEASON	PRODROME	MORPHOLOGY
Viral Causes				
Measles (rubeola virus)	Infants to young adults	Winter/spring	High fever, signs and symptoms of upper respiratory tract infection, conjunctivitis	Erythematous macules and papules become confluent
Rubella (rubella virus)	Adolescents/ young adults	Spring	Absent or low-grade fever, malaise	Rose pink papules that are not confluent
Erythema infectiosum (parvovirus B19)	5–15 y	Winter/spring	Usually none	Slapped cheeks: reticulate erythema or maculopapular
Roseola (herpesvirus 6)	6 mo–3 y	Spring/fall	High fever for 3–5 days	Maculopapular rash appears after fever declines
Human immunodeficiency virus	Adults	Any season	Fever, malaise, sore throat, diarrhea	Roseola-like hemorrhagic macules
Chickenpox (varicella-zoster virus)	1–14 y	Late fall/ winter/spring	Usually none	Macules, papules rapidly become vesicles on erythematous base, then crusts
Enteroviral exanthems (coxsackie viruses, echo viruses, other enteroviruses)	Young children	Summer/fall	Fever (occasional)	Extremely variable; maculopapular, petechial, purpura, vesicular
Epstein-Barr exanthems (Epstein-Barr virus)	Young children/ adolescents	Any season	Fever, adenopathy, sore throat	Maculopapular or morbilliform
Gianotti-Crosti syndrome (hepatitis B, coxsackie virus infection, Epstein-Barr virus, etc.)	1–6 y	Any season	Usually absent	Papules/paulovesicles; may become confluent
Bacterial and Rickettsial Causes				
Staphylococcal scalded skin syndrome (*S. aureus*/ epidermolytic toxin)	Neonates and infants	Any season	None	Abrupt onset, tender erythroderma
Toxic shock syndrome (staphylococcal toxin)	Adolescents/ young adults	Any season	None	Macular erythroderma
Scarlet fever (*β-Streptococcus*)	School-age children	Fall to spring	Acute onset with fever, sore throat	Diffuse erythema with sandpaper texture
Meningococcemia (meningococcus)	<2 y	Winter/spring	Malaise, fever, upper respiratory tract infection symptoms	Papules, petechiae, purpura
Rocky mountain spotted fever (*Rickettsia rickettsii* carried by ticks)	Any age	Summer	Fever, malaise	Maculopapular/petechial rash
Unknown Cause				
Kawasaki disease (etiology unknown)	6 mo–6 y	Winter/spring	Irritability	Polymorphous-papular, morbilliform, erythema with desquamation

(From Howard R, Frieden IJ: Viral exanthems. In Arndt KA, LeBoit PE, Robinson JK, Wintroub BU [eds]: Cutaneous Medicine and Surgery. WB Saunders, Philadelphia, 1996, with permission.)

DISTRIBUTION	ASSOCIATED FINDINGS	DIAGNOSIS	SPECIAL MANAGEMENT
Begins on face and moves downward over whole body	Koplik's spots, toxic appearance, photophobia, cough, adenopathy, fever	Clinical; acute/convalescent hemagglutinin serology	Report to public health. Oral vitamin A therapy
Begins on face and moves downward	Postauricular and occipital adenopathy; headache, malaise	Rubella IgM or acute/convalescent hemagglutinin serology	Report to public health; check for exposure to pregnant women
Usually arms/legs; may be generalized	Rash waxes/wanes several weeks; occasional arthritis, headache, malaise	Usually clinical; acute/convalescent serology	
Trunk, neck; may be generalized; lasts hours to days	Cervical and postauricular adenopathy	Usually clinical	
Upper body predominates, palm, soles	Adenopathy	Acute and convalescent HIV-1 serologies	Counseling, referral for consideration of antiviral therapy and follow-up
Often begins on scalp/face; more profuse on trunk than extremities	Pruritic, fever, oral	Usually clinical; Tzanck prep, direct immunofluorescence or viral culture	Antihistamines for itching; aspirin contraindicated (Reye's syndrome); acyclovir
Usually generalized, may be acral	Low-grade fever; occasional myocarditis, aseptic meningitis, pleurodynia, malaise	Usually clinical; viral culture from throat, rectal swabs in selected cases	If petechiae or purpura, must consider meningococcemia
Trunk, extremities	Cervical adenopathy Liver/spleen enlarged	Mono spot; Epstein-Barr nuclear antigen acute/convalescent; IgG-viral capsid antigen	
Face, arms, legs, buttocks, spares torso	Occasional lymphadenopathy, hepatomegaly, splenomegaly	Clinical, hepatitis B and Epstein-Barr serologies when indicated	
Diffuse with perioral, perinasal scaling	Fever, conjunctivitis rhinitis	Clinical; culture of S. aureus from systemic site (not skin)	Neonate: if blistering present, hospitalize for intravenous nafcillin and fluid/electrolyte therapy
Generalized	Hypotension; fever, myalgias, diarrhea/vomiting	Clinical case definition criteria isolation S. aureus cervix, etc.	Treatment of hypotension, admit to hospital; antibiotics to eradicate S. aureus
Facial flushing with circumoral pallor, linear erythema in skin folds	Exudative pharyngitis, palatal petechiae, abdominal pain	Throat culture	Penicillin, intramuscularly or orally Penicillin or erythromycin
Trunk, extremities, palms, soles	Temp > 40°C	Clinical blood culture, spinal tap	Immediate intravenous penicillin in emergency department, treatment for shock, if present
Wrists, ankles, palms, soles; trunk later	Central nervous system, pulmonary, cardiac lesions	Serology	Treat on presumptive clinical grounds
Generalized, often with perineal accentuation	Conjunctivitis, cheilitis, glossitis, peripheral edema, adenopathy	Clinical	Admit to hospital for intravenous gamma globulin, salicylates

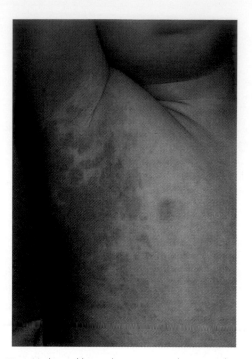

Figure 19.1 Unilateral laterothoracic exanthem—a distinctive exanthem of unknown etiology.

Clinical Features

Most cases in the United States occur in infants less than 15 months of age, with a second peak in incidence in adolescence. The disease is most prevalent in winter and spring. It is spread via droplets from respiratory secretions. The incubation period is from 9 to 12 days from the time of exposure to the onset of symptoms.[3]

Three clinical forms of measles have been described: typical measles, modified measles, and atypical measles. In *typical measles,* the prodrome lasts from 2 to 4 days. Fever as high as 38.5° to 40°C, nasal congestion, sneezing, rhinitis, conjunctivitis, and cough are nearly always present. A transitory macular or urticarial rash has been described early in the prodrome. Koplik's spots, virtually pathognomonic of measles, develop during the prodrome, consisting of tiny white or bluish-gray specks approximately 1 mm in size, superimposed on an erythematous, granular base, beginning on the buccal mucosa, opposite the lower molars, then spreading to involve other parts of the buccal mucosa and to the palate (Fig. 19.2). The pharynx is frequently injected. The measles exanthem usually appears 3 to 5 days after the onset of the prodrome, approximately 14 days after viral exposure. At this time, Koplik's spots are virtually always present, although they begin to fade over the next 3 days. The rash of measles begins behind the ears and at the hairline (Fig. 19.3). The rash spreads centrifugally from head to foot, so that by the third day of the rash, the whole body is involved. Lesions begin as discrete, erythematous papules, which gradually coalesce (Fig. 19.4). They are occasionally purpuric, but pruritus is uncommon. The rash fades after 3 to 4 days but may persist for 6 to 7 days.[3–5]

Complications, more common in developing countries and in immunocompromised hosts, include pneumonia, otitis media, laryngotracheobronchitis, encephalitis, myocarditis, and pericarditis. "Black measles," a rare form of measles, is characterized by the abrupt onset of fever and delirium, followed by respiratory distress and an extensive confluent hemorrhagic eruption resembling disseminated intravascular coagulation. Infection during pregnancy is associated with a high incidence of fetal wastage and, in some cases, congenital malformations.

Modified measles usually occurs in partially immune hosts, such as infants younger than 9 months of age and in cases where partial vaccine failure has occurred. The prodrome may be shortened, and cough, congestion, and fever may be less severe. The presence of Koplik's spots is variable. The skin eruption is usually less confluent. In recent epidemics, many cases of measles were probably missed because of atypical presentations.

Atypical measles is rarely seen because it occurred mainly in individuals previously vaccinated with killed-measles virus vaccine. The main characteristics are fever, onset of an acrally-located hemorrhagic rash, and pneumonia.

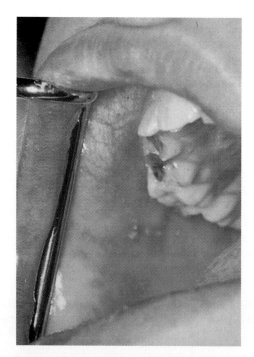

Figure 19.2 Koplik's spots. (Courtesy of University of Iowa, Department of Dermatology.)

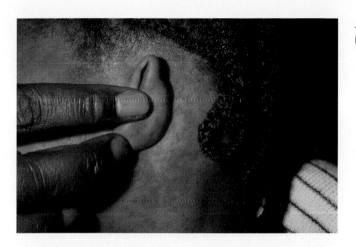

Figure 19.3 Measles begins behind the ears and at the hairline. (From Frieden and Penneys,[4] with permission.)

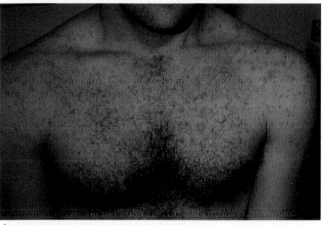

Figure 19.4 (A & B) 31-year-old adult male with measles.

A

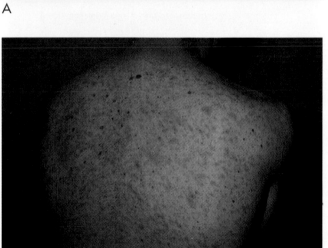

B

Pathology

Biopsies of skin lesions are rarely, if ever, necessary but may demonstrate parakeratosis, dyskeratosis, spongiosis, and syncytial giant cells.

Diagnosis

The diagnosis of measles is usually clinical but can be confirmed with acute and convalescent serology for hemagglutination inhibition or measles IgM. Virus may be isolated from the blood, respiratory tract, skin, and other organs.

Treatment

High-dose oral vitamin A significantly decreases the morbidity and mortality in hospitalized children with measles. Retinyl palmitate is given in a dosage of 400,000 IU in two divided doses separated by 24 hours. The American Academy of Pediatrics has recommended this treatment for all children aged 6 months to 2 years hospitalized with measles, as well as those of other ages with immunodeficiency, ophthalmologic evidence of vitamin A deficiency, or moderate to severe malnutrition including impaired intestinal absorption and in recent immigrants from areas with high mortality rates from measles. No specific antiviral therapy is available.[6]

Differential Diagnosis

Typical measles usually is not difficult to distinguish from other childhood exanthems, especially early in the course of infection, when Koplik's spots are present, but it may be confused with drug eruptions and other exanthems, particularly Kawasaki disease. Atypical measles may be exceedingly difficult to differentiate from Rocky Mountain spotted fever.

RUBELLA

Infection with rubella usually causes a mild illness with exanthem. The most feared complication is the severe congenital infection that may result from infection during pregnancy. Rubella was once a common cause of exanthem, but it has become rare following widespread use of the rubella vaccine. The majority of cases now occur in individuals over the age of 15, primarily because of failure to be vaccinated.[3,6]

Etiology

Rubella is caused by the rubella virus, an RNA virus that is a member of the Togaviridae family.

Clinical Features

Rubella occurs most commonly in the spring. After an incubation period of 15 to 21 days, a prodrome of malaise, cough, sore throat, fever, headache, and eye pain occurs. The rash can be variable in both extent and duration. Discrete pink macules and papules begin on the face and progress downward to involve the trunk and extremities (Fig. 19.5). The rash may become confluent and at times may appear morbilliform or even scarlatiniform. An enanthem (Forschheimer spots) consisting of pinpoint rose-colored macules and petechiae on the soft palate occasionally occurs. Adenopathy is prominent, particularly of the suboccipital and postauricular regions. Fever is usually mild or absent. Arthritis and arthralgias are most common in women.

Diagnosis

The white blood count is often low, with neutropenia. Hemagglutination inhibition is commonly used for

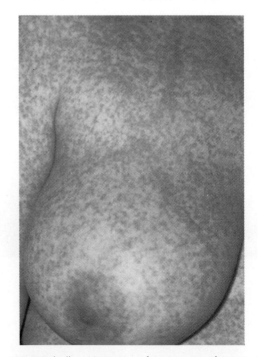

Figure 19.5 Rubella. (Courtesy of University of Iowa, Department of Dermatology.)

diagnosis. Positive rubella-specific IgM indicates acute infection and may be helpful in clinical settings where pregnant women are involved. A fourfold rise in hemagglutination inhibition/IgG is also diagnostic of rubella.[6]

Treatment

There is no specific treatment.

Differential Diagnosis

The differential diagnosis includes other exanthems, especially those caused by measles and enteroviruses.

ROSEOLA

Roseola (exanthema subitum) is one of the most common childhood exanthems. It is characterized by a febrile illness of 3 to 5 days' duration, followed by an abrupt decrease in fever and then by the appearance of the exanthem.

Etiology

Recent studies strongly suggest that the disease is caused by human herpesvirus 6 (HHV-6) and can also be caused by human herpesvirus 7.[7,8]

Clinical Features

Virtually all cases of roseola occur between 6 months and 3 years of age in 95% of cases, with 55% occurring in the first year of life. The age of infection is probably explained by acquisition of infection from previously infected asymptomatic individuals who shed the virus from saliva. Most cases are sporadic, and there is no strong seasonal variation to the illness. The incubation period is 5 to 15 days.

Although a prodrome of high fever for 3 to 5 days has been virtually a requirement for diagnosis, cases of acute HHV-6 infection without fever have now been documented. Affected infants generally appear well but may have mild irritability or malaise. Mild upper respiratory symptoms, adenopathy, pharyngitis, tonsillitis, and an enanthem of tiny pink papules on the uvula and soft palate may also be present. The fever decreases abruptly, and a few hours to 2 days later a rash appears, which without the characteristic febrile prodrome is quite nonspecific in its morphology. Rose-pink macules and maculopapules 2 to 5 mm in size and somewhat irregular in configuration appear, most commonly on the neck and trunk (Fig. 19.6). Their duration is usually brief, from a few hours to 1 or 2 days. Pruritus and desquamation are uncommon. Complications of roseola are rare but include febrile seizures, encephalitis, and thrombocytopenic purpura. HHV-6 infection has also been implicated as a cause of a mononucleosis-like syndrome in adults.[4]

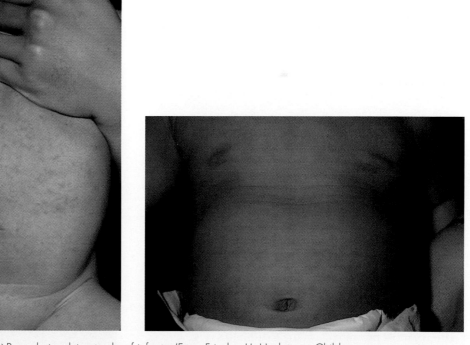

Figure 19.6 *(A & B)* Roseola-involving trunks of infants. (From Friedan IJ: Update on Childhood Exanthems. In: Dahl MV, Lynch P [eds]: Current Opinion in Dermatology. Current Science, Philadelphia, 1993, with permission.)

Diagnosis

Documentation of HHV-6 infection via polymerase chain reaction or acute and convalescent titers is available in research settings only.

Treatment

In vitro data suggest that HHV-6 is sensitive to ganciclovir and foscarnet, but these potentially toxic drugs should be reserved for cases with severe complications.

Differential Diagnosis

The differential diagnosis of the rash includes other viral exanthems and drug eruptions.

ERYTHEMA INFECTIOSUM

Etiology

Erythema infectiosum (fifth disease) is caused by human parvovirus B19 infection. This virus is also recognized as a cause of transient aplastic crisis in patients with hemolytic anemias and hemoglobinopathies, of chronic anemia in immunodeficient patients, and of an arthritis similar to rheumatoid arthritis. It can also result in intrauterine infection and fetal death in infected pregnant women.

Clinical Features

The virus can affect all age groups, but the classic exanthem, erythema infectiosum, is most common in school-aged children, aged 5 to 15. The incubation period is usually between 4 and 14 days but may last as long as 20 days. The disease is transmitted via respiratory secretions.[3,9]

In its classic form, erythema infectiosum is characterized by the sudden onset of rash, which sometimes follows a mild prodrome consisting of low-grade temperature, malaise, and headache. The fiery red rash on the cheeks, so-called slapped cheeks, can be either macular erythema or slightly raised edematous plaques (Fig. 19.7). One to 4 days later a more generalized rash develops, beginning as discrete erythematous macules and papules but gradually evolving into a distinctive lacy, reticular pattern, most prominent on the extremities (Fig. 19.8). This rash waxes and wanes for up to several weeks, perhaps exacerbated by temperature changes, exercise, sunlight exposure, and emotional factors.

Parvovirus B19 also causes less distinctive exanthems. In one documented epidemic, only 50% of patients had a facial rash, and only 1 of 15 patients had the classic slapped-cheek appearance or lacy reticular rash on the extremities. Others had more nonspecific maculopapular eruptions, lasting from 1 to 30 days, with an average of 7.8 days.

Patients with erythema infectiosum typically feel well, but constitutional symptoms such as headache, fever, sore throat, and coryza occur in 5 to 15% of children. Arthritis is the most common complication in adults but is relatively rare in children.

Diagnosis

Diagnosis can be made with parvovirus-specific IgM or acute and convalescent IgG titers. Other assays include direct detection of B19 DNA by nucleic acid hybridization, which is the most sensitive test method of detection.[3,9]

Treatment

No specific antiviral treatment or vaccine for erythema infectiosum is available. Patients with hematologic complications of infection have been successfully treated with intravenous γ-globulin.

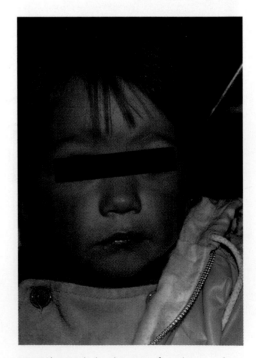

Figure 19.7 "Slapped cheek" sign of erythema infectiosum.

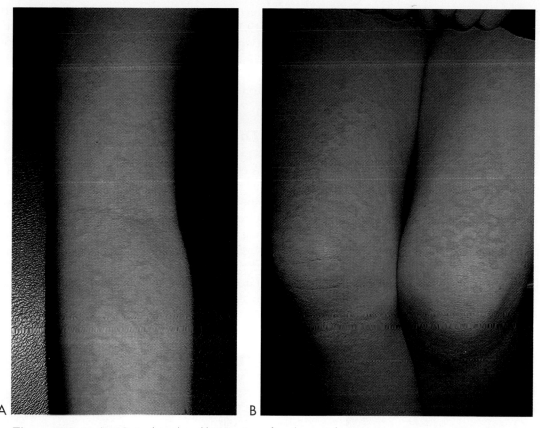

Figure 19.8 (A & B) Reticulate, lace-like eruption of erythema infectiosum.

Diagnosis

The differential diagnosis includes other viral exanthems.

When arthritis is present along with the rash, juvenile rheumatoid arthritis must be considered in the differential diagnosis.

ENTEROVIRAL EXANTHEMS

Enteroviruses are the leading cause of childhood exanthems in the summer and fall.

Etiology

This family of viruses was originally subdivided into three separate groups—poliovirus, coxsackievirus, and echovirus—but the discovery of viruses with antigenic properties common to more than one group led to reclassification. Those previously designated as echovirus, coxsackievirus, or poliovirus have retained these names, but newly recognized enteroviruses are labeled enterovirus 68, 69, and so on.

Clinical Features

These viruses are responsible for a wide array of clinical syndromes, and over 30 of them cause exanthems. They are spread by the fecal-oral route. The incubation period is usually 3 to 5 days.[3]

The cutaneous manifestations of enteroviral infections are quite pleomorphic. Rubelliform, morbilliform, roseola-like, scarlatiniform, urticarial, pustular, petechial, purpuric, and hemangioma-like eruptions have all been described. Infection is most common in August, September, and October and may account for up to two-thirds of all summer exanthems.

Age at the time of infection appears to influence the clinical manifestations. Exanthems are much more common in young children, whereas central nervous system involvement is more common in older children. Most enteroviral exanthems other than hand-foot-and-mouth disease are not distinctive enough to allow for specific clinical diagnosis, but time of year, morphology, and associated findings, such as aseptic meningitis, pleurodynia, and myocarditis, may aid in diagnosis.

Echovirus 9 is a very prevalent enterovirus, and several thousand cases have been studied. The rash is most commonly maculopapular, beginning on the face and spreading to the body. A petechial rash may occur and, because infection may be associated with aseptic meningitis, can mimic meningococcemia.[3]

Hand-foot-and-mouth-disease is one of the most characteristic syndromes caused by enteroviruses and has been reported with multiple enteroviruses including coxsackievirus A16 (most commonly) as well as coxsackievirus A5, A7, A9, A10, B2, B3, B5 and enterovirus 71. A brief prodrome of low-grade fever, anorexia, malaise, and sore throat is followed by the onset of the characteristic enanthem. Lesions in the mouth begin as vesicles but rapidly erode, developing into sharply marginated ulcers, which vary in size from a few millimeters to 2 cm. Common locations include the buccal mucosa and tongue, but the palate, uvula, and anterior tonsillar pillars are often affected (Fig. 19.9).

An exanthem is present in the majority of cases. Gray-white angulated or round vesicles, ranging in size from 3 to 7 mm, are most prominent on the dorsal hand and feet but may also occur on the palms and soles (Fig. 19.10). The diaper area is often affected in young infants (Fig. 19.11). A more generalized maculopapular or vesicular rash is occasionally present. Pain and itching are variable, and the rash may be completely asymptomatic.[10]

Diagnosis

A clinical diagnosis of enterovirus exanthem is sufficient in most cases, without confirming laboratory tests. If specific diagnosis is needed, the best method is viral culture. Collection of specimens from multiple sites including the stool, pharynx, urine, and cerebrospinal fluid increases the likelihood of recovering the virus. Acute and convalescent serologies may be helpful if a specific enterovirus is suspected, but the large number of serotypes makes serologic diagnosis impractical in most cases.

Figure 19.9 Oral lesions of hand-foot-and-mouth syndrome.

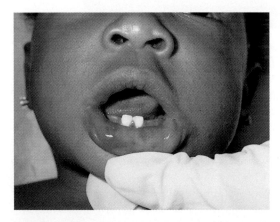

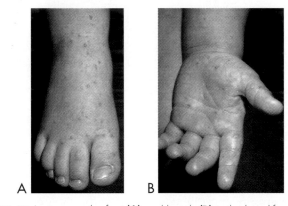

A   B

Figure 19.10 Lesions on the feet **(A)** and hands **(B)** in the hand-foot-and-mouth syndrome. (Fig. A from Frieden and Resnick,[10] with permission; Fig. B from Frieden and Penneys,[4] with permission.)

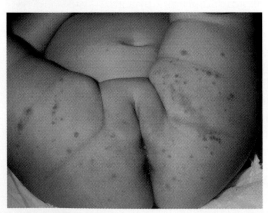

Figure 19.11 Buttock lesions of hand-foot-and-mouth syndrome. (From Frieden and Penneys,[4] with permission.)

Treatment

No specific therapy is available for enteroviral infections. Enteric precautions are recommended in hospitalized patients.[3]

Differential Diagnosis

Because of the wide array of clinical manifestations, a number of other infectious exanthems must be considered. When purpura is present, it may include meningococcemia, whereas when vesicular exanthems are present, it mimics varicella.

EPSTEIN-BARR VIRUS INFECTION

Clinical Features

Exanthems due to Epstein-Barr virus (EBV) infection occur most commonly in three clinical settings. Generalized rashes occur in up to 35% of young children with acute EBV infection. The morphology may be maculopapular, scarlatiniform, papulovesicular, or erythema multiforme–like (Fig. 19.12). Associated findings include fever, upper respiratory tract congestion, adenopathy, and hepatosplenomegaly. A distinctive rash may also occur following administration of ampi-

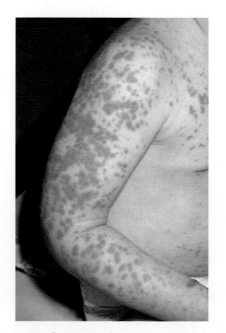

Figure 19.12 Confluent papular eruption due to Epstein-Barr virus infection.

cillin or other antibiotics to older children and adults with mononucleosis due to EBV. Erythematous macules and papules begin on the trunk and may spread over the entire body, becoming confluent in some areas. EBV infection can also cause Gianotti-Crosti syndrome (see below).

Diagnosis

Laboratory findings depend on the age at the time of infection. The monospot test is frequently negative in children less than 4 years of age. In these cases, IgG to the viral capsid antigen is usually detectable at the time of examination. Early antigen antibodies appear weeks to months after onset of infection and may correlate with severe, protracted disease. EBV nuclear antigen appears 3 to 4 weeks after onset of the disease and persists for life.[11]

Differential Diagnosis

Other exanthems and drug eruptions may mimic EBV exanthems.

GIANOTTI CROSTI SYNDROME

The Gianotti-Crosti syndrome is an exanthem characterized by erythematous papular rashes affecting primarily the face and extremities, with relative sparing of the chest, abdomen, and back. In 1955, Gianotti and Crosti described a distinctive eruption characterized by the presence of multiple, discrete, nonpruritic, erythematous papules located exclusively on the face, neck, and extremities. They later discovered that this rash, which they called "papular acrodermatitis of childhood," was due to hepatitis B. It is now appreciated that many other infectious agents can cause similar rashes. The forms caused by other agents have sometimes been called "papulovesicular acro-located syndrome" to distinguish them from the hepatitis B–associated exanthem, but the term "Gianotti-Crosti syndrome" is also used.[12,13]

Etiology

Most cases of Gianotti-Crosti syndrome are due to EBV, cytomegalovirus, and enteroviruses, but cases due to poliovirus, hepatitis A, parainfluenza virus, and of course hepatitis B have been reported.[12,13]

Clinical Features

The age of affected children varies from 3 months to 15 years, with a peak incidence at 2 to 5 years of age. Both sexes are affected equally. Most cases associated with hepatitis B infection, are due to the AYW subtype, but this is now an uncommon cause, even in Italy, where it was originally described.

The distribution of Gianotti-Crosti syndrome is distinctive and usually the first clue to diagnosis. Whereas most exanthems have significant involvement of the torso, this syndrome spares the torso, with most lesions being noted on the face and extremities, with occasional involvement of the buttocks. Lesions may vary from flat-topped papules to juicy, papulovesicular lesions resembling insect bites (Fig. 19.13). Pruritus is variable. Hepatomegaly and lymphadenopathy may be present, depending on the etiology. The rash persists longer than most exanthems, often lasting from 2 to 4 weeks.

Diagnosis

The diagnosis is usually made clinically. Evaluation of children with papular, acrally located eruptions should include a history of exposure to hepatitis and other infectious illnesses. Evaluation should include a careful examination for lymphadenopathy, hepatomegaly, and splenomegaly. If an exposure history suggests the possibility of hepatitis B infection, laboratory evaluation including a complete blood count, liver function tests, and hepatitis B surface antigen should be obtained. Because any hepatitis B is quite rare in the United States, such serologic testing is probably not necessary in all cases.

Treatment

There is no specific treatment. Oral antihistamines are occasionally necessary. The prognosis is generally good,

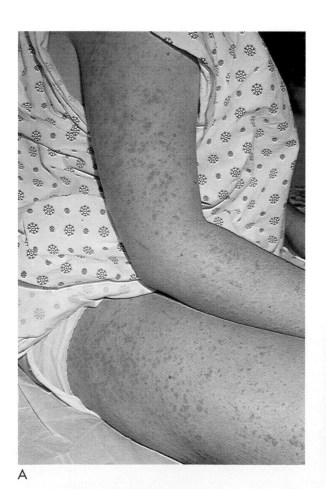
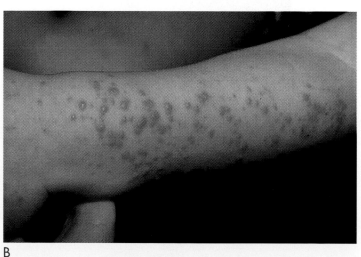

A

B

Figure 19.13 (A & B) Gianotti-Crosti syndrome. (From Frieden and Resnick,[10] with permission.)

although some children with hepatitis B–associated disease go on to develop chronic hepatitis.

Differential Diagnosis

The differential diagnosis includes papular urticaria, erythema multiforme, and frictional lichenoid dermatitis. A skin biopsy is occasionally necessary to differentiate the condition from other papular eruptions of childhood. Most cases show a spongiotic dermatitis, with a variable degree of superficial and deep lymphocytic infiltration. More well-developed lesions may have psoriasiform epidermal hyperplasia and occasionally marked edema of the papillary dermis.

REFERENCES

1. McCuaig CC, Russo P, Powell J et al: Unilateral laterothoracic exanthem: a clinicopathologic study of forty-eight patients. J Am Acad Dermatol 34:979, 1996

2. Goodyear HM, Laidler PS, Price EH, Kenny PA, Harper JI: Acute infectious erythemas in children: a clinico-microbiologic study. Br J Dermatol 124:433, 1991

3. Feigin RD, Cherry JD: (eds): Textbook of Pediatric Infectious Diseases. 3rd Ed. WB Saunders, Philadelphia, 1992

4. Frieden IJ, Penneys NS: Viral infections. p. 1257. In Schachner LA, Hansen RC (eds): Pediatric Dermatology. 2nd Ed. Churchill Livingstone, New York, 1995

5. Hogan PA, Morelli JG, Weston WL: Viral exanthems. Curr Probl Dermatol 4:43, 1992

6. Committee on Infectious Diseases, American Academy of Pediatrics 1994 Red Book: Report of the Committee on Infectious Diseases. 23rd Ed. American Academy of Pediatrics, Elk Grove Village, IL, 1994

7. Asano Y, Yoshikawa T, Suga S et al: Clinical features of infants with primary human herpesvirus 6 infection (exanthem subitum, roseola infantum). Pediatrics 93:104, 1994

8. Torigoe S, Kumamoto T, Koide W, Taya K, Yamanishi K: Clinical manifestations associated with human herpesvirus 7 infection. Arch Dis Child 72:518, 1995

9. CDC: Risks associated with human parvovirus B19 infection. MMWR 38:81, 1989

10. Frieden IJ, Resnick SD: Childhood exanthems: old and new. Pediatr Clin North Am 38:859, 1991

11. Sumaya CV, Ench Y: Epstein-Barr virus infectious mononucleosis in children: I. Clinical and general laboratory findings. II. Heterophil antibody and viral-specific responses. Pediatrics 75:1003, 1985

12. Caputo R, Gelmetti C, Ermacora E, Gianni E, Silvestri A: Gianotti-Crosti syndrome: a retrospective analysis of 308 cases. J Am Acad Dermatol 26:207, 1992

13. Draelos ZK, Hansen RC, James WD: Gianotti-Crosti syndrome associated with infections other than hepatitis B. JAMA 256:2386, 1986

14. Howard R, Frieden IJ: Viral exanthems. In: Cutaneous Medicine and Surgery. An Integrated Program in Dermatology. WB Saunders, Philadelphia, 1996

CHAPTER 20

Antiviral Therapy for Cutaneous Viral Infections

Karl R. Beutner

SUMMARY

Herpes Simplex Virus

Varicella-Zoster Virus

Human Papillomavirus

Molluscum Contagiosum Virus

Psychosocial Issues of Treating Genital Viruses

Treatment of Nongenital Warts

New Treatments: Therapeutic Implants, Cidofovir, Imiquimod, Vaccines

This chapter focuses on the practical treatment of cutaneous viral infections. The prospective placebo-controlled study is the mainstay for our understanding of the treatment of these infections. Because of the wide spectrum of disease produced by these viruses, it is not possible to conduct a trial for every clinical presentation. Readers are urged to blend the comments in this chapter with their experience and other readings with the goal to be consistent and rational in the treatment of these infections. Learning how to use antiviral drugs is an evolutionary process. Little more than a decade ago, the prospect of safe, effective antiviral therapy was remote. This area is clearly dynamic and ever changing.

The viruses that commonly replicate in the epidermis include herpes simplex virus (HSV) types 1 and 2, varicella-zoster virus (VZV), human papillomavirus (HPV), molluscum contagiosum virus (MCV), and enteroviruses. Since cutaneous viral infections are only rarely fatal, the key to treatment is understanding the natural history of the condition being treated. Not every cutaneous viral infection needs to be treated. In the area of herpes infection, modern treatment has focused primarily on the use of antiviral agents. Newer approaches in the form of vaccines and immune enhancers will attempt to exploit natural immune responses that normally control these infections in most patients. Similarly, HPV and MCV are traditionally treated, primarily with ablative modalities, but mainstream therapy may soon change to vaccines and immune enhancers to address the primary event and infection, not the symptom—a bump.

HERPES SIMPLEX VIRUS

The HSV group represents an epidermotrophic virus, which most commonly infects the lips and genital area but can infect any cutaneous site. HSV infection of the hand produces herpetic whitlow. Extensive HSV infection of preexisting skin diseases can result in eczema herpeticum or Kaposi's varicelliform eruption. HSV infection of the arm and trunk is often referred to as herpes gladiatorum because it can be frequently seen in wrestlers and other atheletes. Conceptually, with any recurrent localized vesiculobullous eruption, HSV infection must be considered in the differential diagnosis.

POTENTIAL OUTCOMES OF GENITAL HERPES SIMPLEX VIRUS INFECTION

Primary episode

> *Patient without oral herpes infected with genital herpes presents in 7–14 days with severe cutaneous and systemic signs and symptoms. This is the least common event.*

Nonprimary first episode

> *Patient presents with first episode of genital herpes months or years after infection. This is usually milder than the primary episode.*

Recurrent genital herpes

> *Either of the above patients can have recurrent episodes.*

Asymptomatic genital herpes

> *The most common outcome of infection (60% of those infected) shed HSV periodically without symptoms and are infectious but do not have recognized outbreaks.*

Everyone infected with HSV will have one of three outcomes. Perhaps the most common event is a person becomes infected and never has a symptomatic outbreak. These individuals may be periodically infectious because of asymptomatic shedding. The second most common outcome is the development of a first recognized outbreak months or years after the acquisition of the virus. This has been referred to as a nonprimary or initial episode, and it tends to be less severe than a primary episode.

The least common outcome of HSV infection is the patient who presents within 2 weeks of infection with a severe cutaneous eruption, most commonly gingivostomatitis in the case of herpes labialis or extensive genital lesions in the case of herpes genitalis. These primary infections are often accompanied by moderate to severe systemic signs and symptoms. Once patients have had a symptomatic outbreak, they are then susceptible to recurrent disease, which varies greatly in terms of frequency and severity. In general, oral-labial HSV is caused by HSV type 1 and genital herpes by type 2. Type 1 genital herpes is increasingly common.

The treatment of HSV can be divided into acute or episodic, suppressive or continuous, and prophylactic treatment. The goal of episodic treatment is to shorten the duration and severity of the signs and symptoms of an outbreak. The goal of suppressive or continuous therapy is to decrease the frequency of outbreaks over months or years, and the goal of prophylaxis is to prevent outbreaks over a short term. Prophylaxis is initiated prior to and continued until after a known flare factor, such as ultraviolet light exposure or stress, is anticipated.

Routes of administration of currently available antiherpetic therapies include topical, oral, and intravenous (Tables 20.1 and 20.2). Topical therapy is of historical interest and, at least with currently available topical agents, should be actively discouraged, primarily because of poor efficacy and the superiority of oral dosage forms. The intravenous route of administration is available but rarely needed for infections limited to the skin in immunocompetent patients, particularly since the second-generation oral antiherpetics have greatly improved bioavailability.

In the episodic treatment of these infections, the goal is to treat moderate to severe disease as early as possible. The patient with recurrent oral or genital herpes with episodes that last 2 to 4 days and mild or no symptoms probably will not benefit from episodic treatment. It is also doubtful that episodic treatment for recurrent disease initiated beyond the first 24 hours is of value, and treatment started after crusting, even for severe disease, will probably not be beneficial.

For a decade, the only available treatment for HSV was acyclovir. There is now the second-generation antiherpetics valacyclovir and famciclovir. Both of these

Table 20.1 Dosages of Antiherpetic Therapies

INFECTION	DOSAGE
Herpes simplex virus	
Episodic therapy of primary or recurrent disease	Acyclovir, 200 mg 5 × a day × 7 days or 400 mg tid × 7 days
	Valacyclovir, 500 mg bid × 7 days
	Famciclovir, 250 mg bid × 7 days
Continuous or suppressive therapy[a]	Acyclovir, 400 mg bid
	Valacyclovir, 500 mg qd
	Famciclovir, 250 mg bid
Varicella zoster virus[b] Primary infection (chickenpox) or recurrent shingles	Children[1]: Acyclovir, 20 mg/kg per dose qid × 5 days, not to exceed 800 mg per dose
	Adults[1]: Acyclovir, 800 mg 5 × a day × 7 days
	Valacyclovir, 1000 mg tid × 7 days
	Famciclovir, 500 mg tid × 7 days

[a] These doses should be considered initial doses; some patients require higher doses, some lower doses. [b] Dosage reduction required for impaired renal function.

new antivirals have oral bioavailability superior to acyclovir with simpler dosing and in some settings greater efficacy. These drugs should replace acyclovir as first-line treatment for cutaneous herpes infections.[1-7]

For reasons that are not totally clear, recurrent herpes labialis appears to be less responsive to antiviral therapy than is recurrent herpes genitalis. For this reason, there appears to be little value in treating mild herpes labialis. What is mild disease? Broadly, it can defined as a cold sore that lasts 2 to 3 days and causes mild or less pain. Moderate to severe cold sores are of longer duration and associated with more symptoms that may benefit from oral antiviral therapy. For primary oral herpes, herpes gingivostomatitis, oral therapy will greatly reduce the signs and symptoms and the duration of infection.

Table 20.2 Currently Available Antiherpetic Drugs

DRUG	ROUTE	DOSAGE	FORM
Acyclovir	Oral	200 mg	Capsules
		400 mg	Caplets
		800 mg	Caplets
		200 mg/5 ml	Suspension
Valacyclovir	Oral	500 mg	Tablets
		1000 mg	Caplets
Famciclovir	Oral	125 mg	Tablets
		250 mg	Tablets

Patients with frequent cold sores will have a dramatic reduction in the number of episodes on suppressive therapy. Controlled trials have demonstrated that acyclovir can be taken prophylactically to prevent ultraviolet-induced cold sores. Therapy should be initiated 1 to 2 days prior to exposure and continued for 1 to 2 days after exposure. Patients should also use a sunscreen-containing lip balm. It may also be beneficial to use short-term prophylactic therapy in other settings, such as the competitive wrestler who has recurrent cold sores and will be excluded from a match if a cold sore is present or individuals who have frequent cold sores associated with stress and would prefer to not have a cold sore for a particular social or professional event.

For genital herpes, careful selection of patients for antiviral therapy is very important (Table 20.3). One of the more effective uses of oral antiviral therapy is the treatment of primary genital herpes. These patients are infected with HSV and present with severe cutaneous lesions and significant systemic signs and symptoms. Unfortunately, these patients are often misdiagnosed or present late in their course. If it is a patient's first episode and vesicles are still present, episodic treatment is justified.

Approximately 20% of the U.S. population are infected with type 2 genital herpes. Of these, 20% are aware of the infection, 20% become aware with education, and 60% have never had a recognized outbreak. Most, if not all of the 20% of HSV-2 seropositive subjects will episodically shed HSV and be infectious. Most infections are transmitted during periods of asymptomatic shedding. These observations have raised two issues: What value is there in episodic treatment, and what strategies can be employed to prevent transmission? The old strategy of preventing transmission by avoiding sexual contact during outbreaks is not effective.

Episodic treatment should decrease the duration of viral shedding as well as local signs and symptoms. As with herpes labialis, mild recurrent herpes genitalis will probably benefit little if any from recurrent antivirals. The clearest benefit is with a moderate to severe recurrent herpes genitalis. Recently, valacyclovir has been shown not only to shorten these episodes but also to abort episodes when patients initiate treatment promptly.

Continuous or suppressive therapy can greatly decrease or prevent recurrent genital herpes and nearly eliminates asymptomatic shedding. However, does continuous antiviral therapy prevent transmission? Traditionally, continuous therapy has been used exclusively for patients with frequent (greater than six per year) outbreaks per year. The frequency of outbreaks should not be the sole criteria for the use of continuous therapy.

INFECTION	ROUTE OF DRUG		
	ORAL	TOPICAL	IV
Herpes labialis			
Primary	+	−	±
Recurrent			
Mild disease	−	−	−
Moderate disease	±	−	−
Severe disease	+	−	−
Suppressive	+	−	−
Prophylactic	+	−	−
Herpes genitalis			
Primary	+	−	+
Recurrent			
Mild disease	−	−	−
Moderate disease	+	−	−
Severe disease	+	−	−
Suppressive	+	−	−
Herpetic whitlow	+	−	−
Eczema herpeticum	+	−	±
Herpes gladiatorum	+	−	−

There are patients with fewer episodes per year but with moderate to severe physical or emotional events associated with each episode. These patients will benefit from a vacation from their herpes. The option for the use of continuous therapy should be reviewed with all patients with recurrent genital herpes.

Other cutaneous HSV infections such as herpetic whitlow, eczema herpeticum, and herpes gladiatorum will benefit from episodic treatment if started promptly. Unfortunately, the challenge with these infections is diagnosis, not treatment.

The discussion thus far has been as it relates to immunocompetent patients; in immunocompromised patients, the frequency and severity of recurrent herpetic infections are much greater. The threshold for treatment should be low, the duration of treatment may need to be longer, and the benefit of treatment is greater.

VARICELLA-ZOSTER VIRUS

Primary infection with VZV results in varicella (chickenpox), while recurrence or reactivation of latent VZV results in zoster (shingles). Because this infection is common and highly infectious, individuals rarely escape their teens without experiencing chickenpox. In general, the severity of primary varicella is inversely related to age, with severity increasing with increasing age. Treatment of chickenpox can significantly reduce the severity of the disease. Treatment should be initiated within the first 24 hours of rash onset.

Zoster or shingles also varies greatly with age. Patients over the age of 50 years are at greater risk of experiencing the complication of chronic pain after zoster, or postherpetic neuralgia. This complication is very rare in patients less than 50 years of age. Antiviral therapy will decrease the duration of viral shedding, accelerate rash healing, and shorten the duration of pain and incidence of postherpetic neuralgia.[8–11]

In patients less than 50 years of age, the primary benefit of treatment is acceleration of rash healing. In patients over 50 years of age, the goal of therapy is not only to speed rash healing but also to have an impact on the duration of pain. The highest-risk patient for chronic pain following zoster is the patient over the age of 60 years with pain before rash (prodromal pain) and moderate or severe pain during the first 3 days. In addition to antiviral therapy, aggressive control of pain early in the course of zoster may shorten the duration of pain. While systemic steroids may improve the quality of life of the zoster patient during the first month or so of infection, they do not have an impact on the frequency of postherpetic neuralgia or the duration of pain. Of patients over the age of 50 who receive antiherpetic therapy, approximately 50% will be pain free by 50 days, 80% will be pain free by 6 months, and less than 1 to 2% will have clinically significant pain beyond 6 months.

HUMAN PAPILLOMAVIRUS

HPV infection results in a broad spectrum of disease as reviewed elsewhere in this volume. Like HSV infection, it appears that most individuals infected with HPV are asymptomatic. When the infection is symptomatic, it manifests on the external genital area as genital warts. External genital warts are defined as warts in the genital area, which includes the penis, scrotum, vulva, urinary meatus, mons pubis, crural folds, perineum, and perianal area, which can be visualized with instrumentation. Treatment of vaginal, intra-anal, intraurethral warts, and cervical HPV infection is beyond the scope of this discussion.

Current treatment of external genital warts provides relief of the symptoms, that is, warts.[12] It is currently unknown if treatment of warts effects infectivity. The treatment of genital warts includes cryotherapy, interferon, podophyllin resin, podofilox, surgery, and trichloroacetic acid (Table 20.4). Scissor excision, electrocautery, thermal coagulation, and laser are the most commonly used surgical modalities. Unfortunately, only intralesional interferon and patient-applied podofilox have been evaluated in prospective, randomized, controlled trials. These treatments may be the least commonly employed modalities, and the most commonly used treatments have not been systematically studied, particularly in terms of standardization, side effects, true efficacy, and recurrence rates.

The choice of treatment modalities is often driven more by what is available in an office or clinic. A major pitfall in the treatment of warts is the repetitive use of a treatment in a patient despite the lack of a clinical response. In general, if there has not been a significant response after three visits, a different modality or referral should be considered, and the need for a biopsy should be evaluated.

There are four morphologic forms of genital warts: (1) condylomata acuminata, or cauliflower-shaped warts, (2) smooth papular warts, (3) keratotic warts, and (4) flat warts. The smooth papular warts can be indistinguishable from bowenoid papulosis or squamous cell carcinoma in situ. Indications for biopsy of genital warts include failure to respond to appropriate therapy, pigmentation (bluish-gray or black), individual warts larger than a thumbnail, or a history of a high-grade cervical lesion in the patient or in a sexual partner of the patient.

Table 20.4 Factors that Should Influence the Selection of Therapy for Genital Warts

THERAPY	WART LOCATION[a]	WART SIZE	TOTAL WART AREA	TOTAL WART COUNT	CLINICIAN EXPERIENCE[c]
Cryotherapy	All sites	Small to average	Limiting[b]	Limiting	+ + + +
Interferon	All sites	All	Limiting	Limiting	+
Podophyllin resin	Moist surfaces	All	Limiting	Not limiting	+
Podofilox	All sites	All	< 10 cm[b]	Not limiting	+
Surgery	All sites/types	All	All	Not limiting	+ + + +
Trichloroacetic acid	Moist surfaces	Small to average	Limiting	Limiting	+

[a] Warts on moist surfaces respond better to some topical treatments than warts on full-keratinized skin.

[b] Treatment of large wart areas or large numbers of warts with certain modalities is too painful and creates wound care problems.

[c] Certain procedures require much greater training and experience.

In selecting treatment, there are a number of important considerations (Table 20.5). There are three types of skin in the genital area: fully keratinized, hair-bearing fully keratinized, non-hair-bearing; and partially keratinized, non-hair-bearing. The surfaces of the last type are often erroneously referred to as mucous membranes because they are moist. They are moist because they are partially keratinized. These areas do not have mucous glands in the dermis or lamina propria.

In general, the condyloma acuminatum type of wart occurs on partially keratinized or moist areas, and papular and keratotic warts occur on fully keratinized areas. The smaller warts on moist surfaces respond well to topical trichloroacetic acid or podophyllin resin, and the warts on dry, keratinized areas respond poorly to these modalities. Other factors that influence treatment selection include wart number, total wart area, anatomic location, clinician's experience, and patient preference. Treatment options should be reviewed with the patient.

Cryotherapy is commonly used but has not been systematically evaluated. Liquid nitrogen is the most common agent used, but the methods of application, such as spray techniques, modified cotton applicator, cryoprobe, and closed cryoprobe systems, are difficult to standardize. A wart cannot be effectively frozen with a tightly wound cotton-tipped applicator used to apply liquid nitrogen. Short of the use of small thermocouples inserted beneath the wart, cryotherapy is difficult to standardize and requires significant training and experience to obtain good results. For reasons that are not clear, local anesthesia is not routinely used with cryotherapy. For more than a few small warts, the use of a topical anesthesia, such as an eutectic mixture of lido-

caine and prilocaine (EMLA) or an injected local anesthetic greatly facilitates cryotherapy.

Intralesional interferon has been well characterized as safe and effective for the treatment of genital warts. However, the demonstrated efficacy is no greater than of other modalities that are far less consumptive of resources. Also, frequent systemic flu-like syndrome associated with intralesional interferon limits its use.

Podophyllin resin is not a caustic but a plant extract with antimitotic activity. While this resin is generally regarded as safe, it has not been standardized, and different preparations vary greatly in their content of active lignins

Table 20.5 Dosage Reduction of Antiviral Therapy for Varicella-Zoster Virus

DRUG	CREATININE CLEARANCE (ml/min)	DOSAGE
Acyclovir	>25	800 mg 5 times a day
	10–25	800 mg tid
	0–10	800 mg bid
Valacyclovir	>25	1,000 mg tid
	30–49	1,000 mg bid
	10–29	1,000 mg qd
	<10	500 mg qd
Famciclovir	>60	500 mg tid
	40–59	500 mg bid
	20–39	500 mg qd

and known and unknown contaminants. The optimum concentration, shelf life, and frequency of application are not known for podophyllin. It is often recommended to apply podophyllin resin in tincture of benzoin and then have the patient wash it off after a few hours. In reality, benzoin is very difficult to remove because it is not water soluble. Used properly, a thin layer of podophyllin should be applied and allowed to dry completely before the patient is returned to a normal anatomic position. Application of excessive amounts that cannot dry will result in the relatively uncontrolled spread of the resin over a wide area and thus significant local reaction.

The major active lignin in podophyllin resin is podofilox (podophyllotoxin), which is commercially available as a 0.5% alcoholic solution or gel for patient application. Patients apply podofilox twice daily for 3 days followed by a 4-day treatment-free period.[13–17] A course of therapy consists of one to six applications of such treatment. Warts on keratinized skin have approximately a 50% complete response rate, while warts on moist surfaces have a response rate approaching 90%. Local reactions are not uncommon but are quite acceptable. Use of podophyllin or podofilox during pregnancy should be avoided.

Surgery has an advantage over other modalities in that the patient is promptly rendered wart free. Surgery has the disadvantage that significant training and experience are required, and some clinicians dislike performing surgery. When done properly, the pain with surgery is less than that produced by cryotherapy or trichloroacetic acid, and scarring is not greater than with other ablative modalities.

Ideally, a topical anesthetic is applied. After 5 to 10 minutes on moist surfaces and 20 to 30 minutes on full keratinized areas, a local anesthetic such as buffered lidocaine is then administered intradermally using a 30-g needle. The local anesthetic also elevates the wart, facilitating a superficial or tangential excision with a fine pair of scissors or a scalpel blade. Warts being epidermal, surgical removal should not be deeper than the upper dermis, ideally limited to the reticular dermis. Hemostasis can then be achieved with a styptic, such as aluminum chloride or very light electrocautery. In addition to gloves, mask, and eye protection, the use of a smoke evacuator should be considered. Wounds heal well in 7 to 14 days. The destruction of tissue is controlled and limited to an area not much larger than the base of the wart. In addition to the above procedures, after local anesthetic is achieved, thermal cautery, loop electrical excision, electrocautery, or laser vaporization can also be used.

The most common caustic agent used to treat genital warts is trichloroacetic acid. This modality is generally regarded as safe and effective but has not been systematically evaluated to determine optimal concentration, frequency of application, efficacy, recurrence rate, and local adverse reactions. In general, 50 to 70% tri-chloroacetic acid is used most frequently and applied every 1 to 2 weeks. As with podophyllin resin, small moist warts appear to be more responsive. If warts have not cleared or significantly improved after three treatments, an alternative therapy should be considered.

There is great variability in the extent of genital warts, but the average patient who has 1 to 10 warts of 0.5 to 1.0 cm^2 in total area is amenable, at least initially, to any of the above treatments. Patient with very large or extensive warts should be referred for appropriate surgical therapy. While patients with large or extensive warts can sometimes respond to topical therapies, it is often a protracted course of therapy.

The goal of therapy is the induction of a wart-free period and the use of a treatment no worse than the disease being treated, as well as prevention or early diagnosis of HPV-related cervical cancer. HPV-associated cancer is not an event that begins with a wart. Patients with genital warts or their sexual partners can be coinfected with oncogenic HPV types. For this reason, women with genital warts or female partners of men with genital warts require cervical cancer screening. The anal canal is also susceptible to the oncogenic potential of HPV. Men and women who have intra-anal warts should be followed carefully for the development of anal cancer, especially if they are immunosuppressed.

Genital warts in immunosuppressed patients are a major problem. Either acquired or iatrogenic immunosuppression will frequently result in not only the development of numerous warts but also in the development of squamous cell carcinoma in some warts on sun-exposed areas. It is important to follow immunosuppressed patients not only to treat the warts but also to monitor them for the development of cutaneous or genital malignancies associated with their HPV infection. In general, the same therapies are applied to their external genital and nongenital warts, although the goals of therapy may be different. In the face of immunosuppression, the major goals of therapy are to try to control the warts so that they do not present a major mechanical or emotional problem and, again, to carefully monitor the patient for the development of HPV-related cutaneous or genital malignancies.

PSYCHOSOCIAL ISSUES

In addition to treatment, patients with genital HSV or HPV infection need education about the natural history of their infection. Without adequate education, these patients often experience significant emotional upset, which influences how they feel about themselves, others, and their sexuality. Effective education requires time and written information.

TREATMENT OF NONGENITAL WARTS

The mainstay of treatment of nongenital warts remains cryotherapy. Other modalities used include surgery, salicylic acid, and immunotherapy with dinitrochlorobenzene. Salicylic acid is particularly useful for plantar warts, remembering that warts, by definition, are confined to the epidermis. The thickness of a wart appears to be dependent on the thickness of the infected epidermis. Thus, warts on the eyelids or genitalia are relatively thin, while warts on the palms and especially the soles of the feet can be very thick. In addition, it is important not to overtreat and create a scar on the sole of the foot, which can produce pain and discomfort for years. An atrophic scar can be sensitive and tender, and a hypertrophic scar can be hard and feel like a rock inside of one's sock.

The chronic moisture such as is produced by hyperhidrosis or chronic vocational or avocational exposure to water may increase the frequency of warts and make them more difficult to treat. If the areas can be kept dry, treatment may be more effective. Treatment of warts on the proximal nail fold should be done carefully, since overaggressive therapy can damage the underlying nail matrix and result in a nail dystrophy. Flat warts on the face and legs represent a number of therapeutic challenges. Shaving of affected areas on men's faces and women's legs can spread the warts. While various concentrations of isotretinoin and 5-fluorouracil are commonly used, there are no studies to support this treatment. With ablative therapy of nongenital warts, in some patients who are in a very active state of wart virus infection, the treatment will result in koebnerization, or worsening of the warts. This can be seen as the production of so-called doughnut warts, where a wart is treated and remains clear but a ring of warts develops around the site that has been treated. When this occurs, consideration should be given to not using further ablative therapies.

MOLLUSCUM CONTAGIOSUM

In the immunocompetent patient, molluscum contagiosum will always resolve without treatment, usually in less than 1 year. Spontaneous resolution is often pre-

---

PITFALLS IN THE TREATMENT OF WARTS

Repetitive ablative therapy to papular lesions that are not warts

Repetitive use of a single ablative therapy to warts failing therapy

Use of a limited number of therapies

Failure to explain therapeutic options, goals of therapy, and potential complications to the patient

---

ceded by an intense inflammatory reaction and sometimes a generalized eruption of small vesiculopapules representing an id reaction.

When treatment is desired, methods most commonly used are superficial curettage, extraction of the molluscum body, cryotherapy, trichloroacetic acid, and electrodesiccation. There are numerous anecdotal reports of topical isotretinoin and a small series on the use of patient-applied podofilox for the treatment of molluscum.

In the immunosuppressed patient, the above modalities are applicable if the patient has relatively few lesions. In the patient with numerous or extensive and frequently recurrent lesions, molluscum contagiosum is very challenging.

NEW TREATMENTS

A therapeutic implant consisting of epinephrine, bovine collagen, and 5-fluorouracil is well into clinical development. Cidofovir (HPMPC) is a nucleotide analog, which applied topically appears to be effective in the cottontail rabbit papilloma model and has had favorable early results in humans. In the area of genital warts, three new therapies are currently under development. Imiquimod is a small molecule capable of enhancing immune responses and stimulating release of cytokines such as interferon and tumor necrosis factor *a*. In clinical trials, topical Imiquimod has a complete response rate as high as 78%, with less than 19% recurrence rate.[18–20] Unlike intralesional interferon, imiquimod does not produce systemic reactions, although local inflammatory reactions are seen.

VACCINES

To date, the greatest success in control of viral infection is achieved with vaccines. Viral vaccines have been given prophylactically to prevent acquisition of infection, and

---

GOALS OF WART THERAPY

Induction of wart-free period

A treatment no worse than the disease

With genital warts, early detection of cervical cancer by appropriate screening

prophylactic vaccines for genital HSV and HPV infection appear to be feasible. The use of vaccines as a therapy, to lessen the severity of disease in patients already infected, appears to be a greater challenge. It is not known what immune response to what viral antigen results in host control of infection. With HPV, it is not known if host control is directed at a viral capsid antigen or wart antigen.

CONCLUSION

With an ever-expanding number of therapies available to treat cutaneous viral infections, there is a need to understand both benefits and limitations of these therapies. Indiscriminate use will not benefit the patients and will not be cost-effective. In general, many of these treatments are underutilized because their proper use is poorly understood.

REFERENCES

1. Sacks SL, Aoki FY, Diaz-Mitoma F et al: Patient-initiated, twice-daily oral famciclovir for early recurrent genital herpes. A randomized, double-blind multicenter trial. Canadian Famciclovir Study Group. JAMA 276:44, 1996

2. Cirelli R, Herne K, McCrary M et al: Famciclovir: review of clinical efficacy and safety. Antiviral Res 29:141, 1996

3. Mertz GJ, Loveless MO, Levin MJ et al: Oral famciclovir for suppression of recurrent genital herpes simplex virus infection in women. A multicenter, double-blind, placebo-controlled trial. Collaborative Famciclovir genital herpes Research Group. Arch Intern Med 157:343, 1997

4. Tyring SK, Douglas JM Jr, Corey L, Spruance SL, Esmann J: A randomized, placebo-controlled comparison of oval valaciclovir and acyclovir in immunocompetent patients with recurrent genital herpes infections. The Valaciclovir International Study Group. Arch Dermatol 134:185, 1998

5. Fife KH, Barbarash RA, Rudolph T, Degregorio B, Roth R: Valacyclovir versus acyclovir in the treatment of first-episode genital herpes infection. Results of an international, multicenter, double-blind, randomized clinical trial. The Valaciclovir International Herpes Simplex Virus Study Group. Sex Transm Dis 24:481, 1997

6. Patel R, Bodsworth NJ, Wolley P et al: Valaciclovir for the suppression of recurrent genital HSV infection: a placebo controlled study of once daily therapy. International Valaciclovir HSV Study Group. Genitourin Med 73:105, 1997

7. Spruance SL, Tyring SK, DeGregorio B, Miller C, Beutner K: A large-scale, placebo-controlled, dose-ranging trial of peroral valaciclovir for episodic treatment of recurrent herpes genitalis. Valaciclovir HSV Study Group. Arch Intern Med 156:1729, 1996

8. Beutner KR, Friedman DJ, Forszpaniak C, Andersen PL, Wood MJ: Valacyclovir compared with acyclovir for improved therapy for herpes zoster in immunocompetent adults. Antimicrob Agents Chemother 39:1533, 1995

9. Tyring S, Barbarash RA, Nahlik JE et al: Famiciclovir for the treatment of acute herpes zoster: effects on acute disease and postherpetic neuralgia. A randomized, double-blind, placebo-controlled trial. Collaborative Famciclovir Herpes Zoster Study Group. Ann Intern Med 123:89, 1995

10. Beutner KR: Valacyclovir: a review of its antiviral activity, pharmacokinetic properties and clinical efficacy. Antiviral Res 28:281, 1995

11. Whitley RJ, Weiss H, Gnann JW et al: Acyclovir with and without prednisone for the treatment of herpes zoster. Ann Intern Med 125:376, 1996

12. Beutner KR, Ferenczy A: Therapeutic approaches to genital warts. Am J Med 102:28, 1997

13. Beutner KR, Conant MA, Friedman-Kien AE et al: Patient-applied podofilox for treatment of genital warts. Lancet 1:831, 1989

14. Greenberg MD, Rutledge LH, Reid R, et al: A double-blind, randomized trial of 0.5% podofilox and placebo for the treatment of genital warts in women. Obstet Gynecol 77:735, 1991

15. Tyring S, Edwards L, Cherry LK et al: Safety and efficacy of 0.5% podofilox gel in the treatment of anogenital warts. Arch Dermatol 134:33, 1998

16. Bonnez W, Elswick RK Jr, Bailey-Farchione A et al: Efficacy and safety of 0.5% podofilox solution in the treatment and suppression of anogenital warts. Am J Med 96:420, 1994

17. Greenberg MD, Rutledge LH, Reid R et al: A double-blind, randomized trial of 0.5% podofilox and placebo for the treatment of genital warts in women. Obstet Gynecol 77:735, 1991

18. Beutner KR, Tyring SK, Trofatter KF Jr et al: Imiquimod, a patient-applied immune-response modifier for treatment of external genital warts. Antimicrob Agents Chemother 42:789, 1998

19. Beutner KR, Spruance SL, Hougham AJ et al: Treatment of genital warts with an immune-response modifier (imiquimod). J Am Acad Dermatol 38:230, 1998

20. Edwards L, Ferenczy A, Eron L et al: Self-administered topical 5% imiquimod cream for external anogenital warts. HPV Study Group. Human Papilloma Virus. Arch Dermatol 134:25, 1998

Index

Note: Page numbers in *italics* indicate figures; page numbers followed by t indicate tables.